ABC OF
HYPERTENSION

D1549339

ABC OF HYPERTENSION

Fourth edition

GARETH BEEVERS

Professor of Medicine
University Department of Medicine, City Hospital, Birmingham, UK

GREGORY Y H LIP

Consultant Cardiologist and Reader in Medicine
University Department of Medicine, City Hospital, Birmingham, UK

EOIN O'BRIEN

Chairman, Blood Pressure Measurement Working Party
British Hypertension Society, Beaumont Hospital, Dublin, Ireland

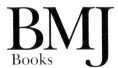

BMJ
Books

© BMJ Books 2001
BMJ Books is an imprint of the BMJ Publishing Group

www.bmjbooks.com

First published in 1981
by the BMJ Publishing Group, BMA House, Tavistock Square,
London WC1H 9JR
First edition 1981
Fifth impression 1985
Second edition 1987
Second impression 1988
Third impression 1988
Fourth impression 1988
Fifth impression 1989
Third edition 1995
Fourth edition 2001
Second impression 2003

British Library Cataloguing in Publication Data
A catalogue record for this book is available from the British Library

ISBN 0-7279-1522-3

Cover design by Marritt Associates, Harrow, Middlesex

Composition by Scribe Design, Gillingham, Kent
Colour reproduction by Tenon and Polert Colour Scanning, Hong Kong
Printed and bound in Spain by GraphyCems, Navarra

Contents

Preface to the fourth edition

The epidemiology, diagnosis and management of hypertension have greatly changed since the first appearance of the *ABC of Hypertension* in the *BMJ* in 1980, and in book form soon afterwards. It was extensively revised in the second and third editions in 1987 and 1995, but the amount of new information since then has necessitated a total re-write for the millennium year. In particular we have attempted to make each chapter more evidence based, with clearly produced tables and figures of the research data on which we have based our recommendations.

The *ABC of Hypertension* is intended to be a clear, practical guide and to provide a basis for greater understanding of the disease, its investigation and its management. The main challenge for clinicians is to ensure that validated treatments are given to all who need them. Since the last edition, the major events that have substantially influenced our management of hypertension include the recognition of new blood pressure targets, the introduction of the angiotensin receptor antagonist group of drugs, and the recognition of the importance of blood pressure control in the management of diabetes mellitus. New chapters in the fourth edition of *ABC of Hypertension* address all these areas. Furthermore, there has been greater integration of the chapters on blood pressure measurement into the clinical management chapters.

We hope that this book will heighten awareness of this common condition, and help improve its management in both hospital and general practice.

Gareth Beevers
Gregory YH Lip
Eoin O'Brien

Abbreviations

TRIALS

AIRE	Acute Infarction Ramipril Efficacy Study
ALLHAT	Antihypertensive and Lipid Lowering Heart Attack Trial
ASCOT	Anglo-Scandinavian Cardiac Outcomes Trial
BHS	British Hypertension Society
CONSENSUS	Co-operative North Scandinavia Enalapril Survival Study
DASH	Dietary Approaches to Stop Hypertension
EWPHE	European Working Party on High Blood Pressure in the Elderly
HAPPHY	Heart Attack Primary Prevention in Hypertension
HDFP	Hypertension Detection and Follow up Programme
HOPE	Heart Outcomes Prevention Evaluation
HOT	Hypertension Optimal Treatment trial
HYVET	Hypertension in the Very Elderly Trial
INSIGHT	International Nifedipine GITS Study Intervention as a Goal in Hypertension Treatment
IPPPSH	International Prospective Primary Prevention Study in Hypertension
JNC-VI	Joint National Committee. Sixth report on hypertension (USA) 1997
LIFE	Losartin Intervention for Endpoints trial
MRC	Medical Research Council
MRFIT	Multiple Risk Factor Intervention Trial
NHA	Nurses Hypertension Association
NHANES	National Health and Nutrition Examination Survey
NORDIL	The Nordic Diltiazem Study
PROGRESS	Perindopril Protection against Recurrent Stroke Study
4S	Scandinavian Simvastatin Survival Study
SAVE	Survival and Ventricular Enlargement Study
SHEP	Systolic Hypertension in the Elderly Program
SOLVD	Studies of Left Ventricular Dysfunction
STOP	Swedish Trial in Old Patients with Hypertension (1 and 2)
SYST-China	Systolic-Hypertension-China trial
SYST-Eur	Systolic Hypertension-Europe trial
TOMHS	Treatment Of Mild Hypertension Study
TSDH	Trials of Systolic and Diastolic Hypertension
UKPDS	United Kingdom Prospective Diabetes Study
USPHS	US Public Health Service Hospital Cooperative Study
VA-1	Veterans Administration

OTHER ABBREVIATIONS

ACE	angiotensin converting enzyme
ARA	angiotensin receptor antagonist
CCB	calcium channel blockers
CHD	coronary heart disease
CVA	cerebrovascular accident (stroke)
CVD	cardiovascular disease
DBP	diastolic blood pressure
IDDM	insulin dependent diabetes mellitus
IDH	isolated diastolic hypertension
ISH	isolated systolic hypertension
LVDD	left ventricular diastolic dysfunction
LVF	left ventricular failure
LVH	left ventricular hypertrophy
LVSD	left ventricular systolic dysfunction
MI	myocardial infarction
MHT	malignant hypertension
NIDDM	non-insulin dependent diabetes mellitus
NNT	number needed to treat
PRA	plasma renin activity
SDH	systolic-diastolic hypertension
SBP	systolic blood pressure

1   Hypertension and cardiovascular risk

Definition of hypertension

Blood pressure has a continuous (bell-shaped) distribution in the population. Thus there are not two separate groups of individuals with and without hypertension but a continuous range of blood pressures from the lowest to the highest, with the majority of individuals falling somewhere in the middle. Using a fairly strict definition of a systolic blood pressure greater than 140 mmHg or a diastolic pressure greater than 90 mmHg or current treatment with antihypertensive medication, the prevalence of hypertension varies from 4% in 18–29 year olds to 65% in the over 80s in the United States population. In some primitive tribal communities, hypertension is virtually unknown.

As the main concern of most clinicians regarding an individual's blood pressure is whether or not it requires treatment, the pragmatic definition of hypertension put forward by the late Professor Geoffrey Rose, that is "that level of blood pressure above which investigation and treatment do more good than harm", would seem to be the most universally acceptable. This level will vary from patient to patient and balances the risks of untreated hypertension with those of long term exposure to antihypertensive drugs and their side effects. It is important to take into account not only the pathological consequences of hypertension but also the psychological and social consequences of labelling a patient as hypertensive, such as difficulties in finding employment and life insurance.

Systolic versus diastolic

There is increasing evidence that the height of the systolic blood pressure is a better predictor of both heart attacks and strokes than the diastolic pressure. Furthermore, the benefits of lowering systolic pressure, when diastolic pressures are not raised, were impressive in the SHEP (Systolic Hypertension in the Elderly Program) and SYST-Eur (Systolic-Hypertension-Europe) studies.

Isolated diastolic hypertension is relatively uncommon and is usually seen in younger patients, so its risk is difficult to quantify. In the Copenhagen City Heart Study the risk from isolated diastolic hypertension was not substantially different from that seen in normotensives, whereas isolated systolic hypertension and systolic-diastolic hypertension were broadly similar (Figure 1.4). This similarity between isolated systolic hypertension and systolic-diastolic hypertension is also seen for left ventricular size, peripheral vascular function, and prothrombotic markers.

- Individuals whose blood pressures are exactly average for the general population are at higher cardiovascular risk than those with lower pressures.
- If a hypertensive patient has a CHD risk of 15% in 10 years then the total cardiovascular risk (i.e. including strokes) rises to 20%.

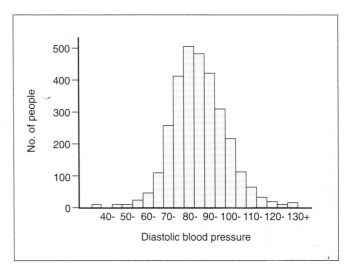

Figure 1.1 Diastolic blood pressure at screening in males in the Renfrew Community Study. Reproduced with permission from Hawthorne VM, Greaves DA, Beevers DG. Blood pressure in a Scottish town. *BMJ* 1974;**3**:600–3.

Table 1.1 Classification of blood pressure for adults aged 18 years and older* Reproduced with permission from The Sixth Report of the Joint National Committee on prevention, detection, evaluation and treatment of high blood pressure (JNC-V1). *Arch Intern Med* 1997;**157**: 2413–46.

Category	Blood pressure (mmHg)		
	Systolic		Diastolic
Optimal†	<120	and	<80
Normal	<130	and	<85
High-normal	130–139	or	85–89
Hypertension‡			
Stage 1	140–159	or	90–99
Stage 2	160–179	or	100–109
Stage 3	≥ 180	or	N ≥ 110

*Not taking antihypertensive drugs and not acutely ill. When systolic and diastolic blood pressures fall into different categories, the higher category should be selected to classify the individual's blood pressure status. For example, 160/92 mmHg should be classified as stage 2 hypertension, and 174/120 mmHg should be classified as stage 3 hypertension. Isolated systolic hypertension is defined as systolic blood pressure 140 mmHg or greater and diastolic blood pressure less than 90 mmHg and staged appropriately (e.g. 170/82 mmHg is defined as stage 2 isolated systolic hypertension). In addition to classifying stages of hypertension on the basis of average blood pressure levels, clinicians should specify pressure levels or absence of target organ disease and additional risk factors. This specificity is important for risk classification and treatment
†Optimal blood pressure with respect to cardiovascular risk is less than 120/80 mmHg. However, unusually low readings should be evaluated for clinical significance
‡Based on the average of two or more readings taken at each of two or more visits after an initial screening

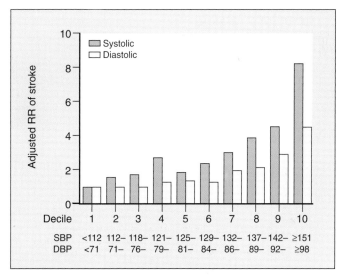

Figure 1.2 Systolic versus diastolic blood pressure and stroke in Multiple Risk Factor Intervention Trial (MRFIT) screenees. Reproduced with permission from Stamler J, Stamler R, Neaton JD. Blood pressure, systolic and diastolic, and cardiovascular risks. US population data. *Arch Intern Med* 1993;**153**:598–615.

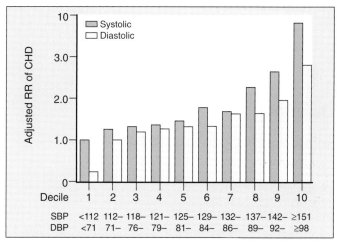

Figure 1.3 The possible impact of a 2 mmHg fall in population average blood pressure on the prevalence of hypertension in the general population and the risk of CHD and strokes. Reproduced with permission from He J, Whelton PK. Elevated systolic blood pressure as a risk factor for cardiovascular and renal disease. *J Hypertens* 1999;**17**(suppl 2):S7–13.

Risks of hypertension

Hypertension is not an uncommon problem. With the increasing age of the general population, the prevalence of hypertension (and its complications) is likely to increase rather than decrease. Many patients will be unaware that they have the condition until they fall victim to its complications of stroke, heart disease, peripheral vascular disease, renal failure, and retinopathy. The detection and treatment of hypertension are therefore vital to reduce cardiovascular disease, strokes, heart failure and renal failure, currently major causes of death in the United Kingdom.

Stroke

Stroke is one of the most devastating consequences of hypertension, resulting not only in premature death but also significant disability. In patients with hypertension about 80% of strokes are ischaemic, caused by intra-arterial thrombosis or embolisation from the heart and large arteries. The remaining 20% are due to various haemorrhagic causes. In the United Kingdom, it is estimated that 40% of all strokes are attributable to systolic blood pressures of 140 mmHg or more. After adjusting for age, men aged 40–59 years with systolic blood pressure at 160–180 mmHg are approximately four-fold at higher risk of stroke during the next 8 years when compared with men with systolic blood pressure at 140–159 mmHg. Data from population studies indicate that an average reduction of just 9/5 mmHg in blood pressure should result in a 34% reduction in the incidence of stroke, whereas a reduction of 19/10 mmHg should result in a 56% lower incidence of stroke.

Hypertension is also associated with an increased risk of atrial fibrillation. The presence of both conditions are additive to the risk of stroke and thromboembolism, with a stroke rate

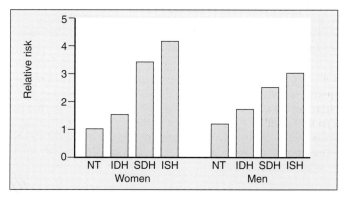

Figure 1.4 Copenhagen City Heart Study-adjusted relative risk of normotensives (NT), isolated diastolic hypertension (IDH), isolated systolic hypertension (ISH), and systolic-diastolic hypertension (SDH). Reproduced with permission from He J, Whelton PK. Elevated systolic blood pressure as a risk factor for cardiovascular and renal disease. *J Hypertens* 1999;**17**(suppl 2):S7–13.

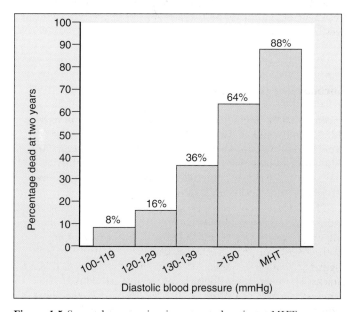

Figure 1.5 Severe hypertension in untreated patients. MHT = malignant hypertension. Data taken from Leishman AWD. Hypertension-treated and untreated: a study of 450 cases. *BMJ* 1959;**1**:1361.

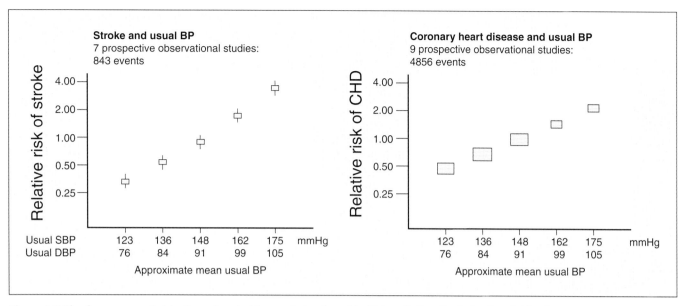

Figure 1.6 Blood pressure and risk. Reproduced with permission from MacMahon S, Peto R, Cutler J *et al*. Blood pressure, stroke and CHD, part 1. Prolonged differences in blood pressure: prospective observational studies collected for the regression dilution bias. *Lancet* 1990;**335**:765–74.

of 8% per year, or more. Interestingly, in the Hypertension Optimal Treatment (HOT) trial, there was no significant reduction in stroke rate by the administration of aspirin. It is possible that this negative finding is due to a preventive effect on cerebral infarction being offset by an increase in cerebral haemorrhage with aspirin.

Dementia

Elderly hypertensives are particularly prone to all forms of stroke and often sustain multiple small, asymptomatic cerebral infarcts, leading to progressive loss of intellectual function and dementia. The recent SYST-Eur study suggested that the treatment of isolated systolic hypertension resulted in the prevention of dementia at follow-up.

Coronary heart disease

Coronary heart disease is six times more common among non-elderly hypertensives than stroke. Adequate treatment of hypertension reduces heart attack risk by approximately 20%, although this analysis is based on blood pressure reduction with the thiazides, calcium channel blockers and beta-blockers, rather than the newer antihypertensive drugs.

There have been recent concerns over the safety of some antihypertensive agents, particularly the short acting dihydropyridine calcium antagonists (such as nifedipine), where a series of pharmacosurveillance case control studies suggested that these agents actually increased the risk of heart attacks. However, recent data from the SYST-Eur trial demonstrated that antihypertensive treatment with the short acting dihydropyridine calcium antagonist, nitrendipine, convincingly reduced strokes and heart attacks, without any increase in conditions previously attributed to the calcium antagonists such as tumours, bleeding and non-cardiac death.

Practice points

- The risk of heart attack and stroke is directly proportional to the height of the blood pressure
- This gradient of risk versus the height of the pressure extends into the usually accepted normal range where the blood pressures are lower than average for western populations
- There is no convincing evidence that, on a long term basis, blood pressures can be too low
- Increasing evidence shows that the systolic blood pressure predicts risk better than the diastolic pressure
- The levels of blood pressure where treatment is worthwhile depend on the clinical trials described in Chapter 2

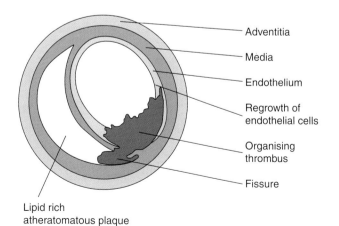

Figure 1.7 Schematic illustration of the process of atheromatous plaque formation, plaque rupture, and thrombus formation, leading ultimately to coronary artery occlusion. From Beevers DG, MacGregor GA. *Hypertension in Practice*. Dunitz: London, 1999.

Left ventricular hypertrophy

As a result of the increased afterload imposed on the heart by high blood pressure, the mass of the left ventricular muscle increases. While this is initially a compensatory response, the increased muscle mass outstrips its oxygen supply and coupled with the reduced coronary vascular reserve seen in hypertension can result in myocardial ischaemia even with normal coronary arteries.

Thus beyond a certain point, left ventricular hypertrophy (LVH) secondary to hypertension becomes a major risk factor for myocardial infarction, stroke, sudden death, and congestive cardiac failure. This increased risk is in addition to that imposed by hypertension itself. In addition, hypertensives with LVH are at increased risk of cardiac arrhythmias (atrial fibrillation, ventricular arrhythmias) and atherosclerotic vascular disease (coronary and peripheral artery disease).

Heart failure

The Framingham study suggested that high blood pressure was the principal cause of heart failure. Those with blood pressures >160/95 mmHg had a six-fold higher incidence of heart failure than those with pressures <140/90 mmHg.

The presence of LVH on the ECG also significantly increased the risk of heart failure. Furthermore, hypertension increases the risk of coronary heart disease, and subsequent myocardial infarction, which can lead to damaged ventricles and heart failure. The development of atrial fibrillation, especially if hypertensive LVH and diastolic dysfunction are present, can precipitate heart failure. Finally, hypertension in association with renal artery stenosis can cause "flash" pulmonary oedema, which can be corrected by treatment of the renal artery stenosis. Nevertheless, heart failure in association with untreated hypertension over many years can slowly be replaced by "normal" blood pressure as the left ventricule progressively fails.

Large vessel arterial disease

Peripheral vascular disease as manifested by intermittent claudication is about three-fold more common in patients with hypertension. Many patients with peripheral vascular disease may also have renal artery stenosis, which may contribute to their hypertension. Atheromatous disease in the aorta coupled with hypertension may progress to aortic aneurysm, the majority of which occur in hypertensives. High pulsatile wave stress and atheromatous disease can lead to dissection of the aortic, which carries a high short term mortality. Extracranial carotid artery disease is also more common in hypertensives.

Renal disease

Renal dysfunction is often found in hypertensives and malignant hypertension frequently leads to progressive renal failure. There is some controversy as to whether mild to moderate essential hypertension leads to renal failure.

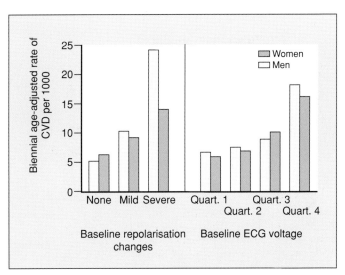

Figure 1.8 Echocardiography of left ventricular hypertrophy in Framingham: 32-year follow-up. Data taken from Post WS, Larson MG, Levy D. Impact of left ventricular structure on the incidence of hypertension. The Framingham Heart Study. *Circulation* 1994;**90**: 179–85. Baseline ECG voltages are divided into quartiles. Repolarisation changes (ST/T depression) are sometimes referred to as "strain".

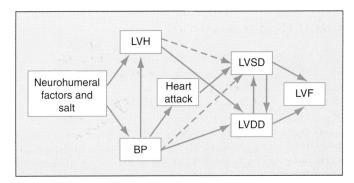

Figure 1.9 The relationships between hypertension, left ventricular hypertrophy (LVH) and left ventricular failure (LVF).

The Keith, Wagener, and Barker classification of hypertensive retinopathy	
Grade 1	Mild narrowing or sclerosis of the retinal arterioles
Grade 2	Moderate to marked sclerosis of the arterioles. Exaggerated arterial light reflex. Arterio-venous nipping
Grade 3	Retinal oedema, cotton wool spots and haemorrhages. Sclerosis and spastic lesions of arterioles. Hard exudates including a macular star
Grade 4	As above and optic disc oedema

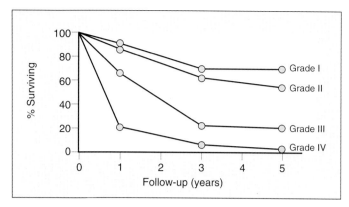

Figure 1.10 Survival curves for retinopathy grades and prognosis in untreated hypertension. Data taken from Keith NM, Wagener HP, Barker NW. Some different types of essential hypertension: their course and prognosis. *Am J Med Sci* 1939;**191**:332–43.

Retinopathy

Hypertension leads to vascular changes in the eye, referred to as hypertensive retinopathy. These changes have been classified by Keith, Wagener and Barker into four grades, which correlate with prognosis. The most severe form of hypertension, that is malignant hypertension, is defined clinically as raised blood pressure in association with bilateral retinal flame shaped haemorrhages, and/or cotton wool spots and/or hard exudates, with or without papilloedema i.e. with grade III or IV retinopathy.

Multiple risk factors

When considering the individual patient it is vital to take other risk factors such as smoking and blood lipids into account. Treating blood pressure alone in the presence of other ongoing risk factors may be relatively ineffective at preventing strokes and myocardial infarction. Coexistent signs of end organ damage also confer a high degree of cardiovascular risk on a patient; for example, left ventricular hypertrophy, previous heart attack, or stroke. However, these may indicate either severity of or late detection of hypertension. Patients with diabetes mellitus have a greatly increased cardiovascular risk, and are discussed in detail in Chapter 11.

Smoking and hyperlipidaemia

The two most important independent risk factors that need to be taken into consideration are smoking and hyperlipidaemia. Data from the MRFIT (Multiple Risk Factor Intervention Trial) trial show that these three risk factors have a synergistic effect. Thus a mildly hypertensive non-smoker with a normal serum cholesterol concentration is a much lower cardiovascular risk than a patient who also smokes and has a raised serum cholesterol concentration.

Recent trials have also established the value of lipid-lowering therapy in primary and secondary prevention of coronary artery disease. While there are no trials of lipid-lowering therapy in uncomplicated essential hypertension, it would be prudent to assess the absolute cardiovascular risk of hypertensives where hyperlipidaemia is also present.

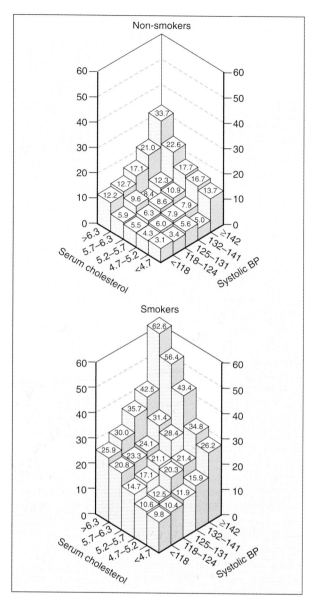

Figure 1.11 The risks of coronary heart disease and stroke in relation to smoking status, serum cholesterol levels and systolic blood pressure mortality per 10 000 person years in the MRFIT screenees. Reproduced with permission from Stamler J, Wentworth D, Neaton JD, for the MRFIT Research Group. Relationship between serum cholesterol and risk of premature death from coronary heart disease: continuous and graded. Findings in 356 222 primary sciences of the Multiple Risk Factor Intervention Trial (MRFIT). *JAMA* 1986;**256**:2823–8.

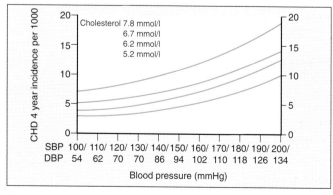

Figure 1.12 The risk of coronary heart disease in relation to hypercholesterolaemia and blood pressure. Four year incidence per 1000 men aged 55 years. Reproduced with permission from Stamler J, Wentworth D, Neaton JD, for the MRFIT Research Group. Relationship between serum cholesterol and risk of premature death from coronary heart disease: continuous and graded. Findings in 356 222 primary sciences of the Multiple Risk Factor Intervention Trial (MRFIT). *JAMA* 1986;**256**:2823–8.

Age

Another factor to take into consideration when deciding about whether to treat hypertension must be the patient's age. Although the relative risk of cardiovascular mortality in a mildly hypertensive young man is raised, the absolute risk of sustaining a stroke or myocardial infarction within the next few years may well be low. However, for an elderly patient with the same degree of hypertension, the absolute risk of stroke or heart attack is much higher as the incidence of these conditions increases with age.

Sex and race

Similarly, women, up to the age of about 50 years, have a lower risk for all levels of blood pressure than men. After the menopause there is a steeper rise in blood pressure when compared to the premenopausal rise of blood pressure with age. Ethnic differences may be important in calculating risk, as hypertension and stroke are particularly common in black people and coronary artery disease is a major cause of death in people originating from the Indian subcontinent.

Public health approach

In contrast to the strategy of assessing a patient's personal risk when making the decision to institute treatment, the public health approach to hypertension would suggest that we should consider community risk, based on the evidence that cardiovascular risk increases with diastolic blood pressure even within the normotensive range. It would seem appropriate to institute education programmes aimed at reducing the blood pressure of the community as a whole.

Shifting the whole bell-shaped curve of diastolic blood pressure distribution 5 mmHg to the left would be associated with an approximately 40% reduction in stroke and a 20–25% reduction in coronary heart disease. Those with very high blood pressures are individually at very high risk of stroke and coronary heart disease but there very few of them, so even if they all had their hypertension perfectly treated it would have very little impact on the number of strokes and heart attacks occurring in the population as a whole. Conversely the majority of strokes and heart attacks occur in those with only mildly elevated or even normal blood pressure. Although it would still seem sensible to identify and treat high risk patients (that is, those with more severe hypertension), the community approach to blood pressure would probably be more cost effective.

There is no evidence of a threshold between "normal" blood pressure and pressure associated with higher risk, and furthermore, very little evidence in untreated populations of a so-called "J-curve", where increased risk might be seen in individuals with low blood pressures. At a population level, a lower level of cardiovascular risk is seen in women, at least below the age of 55 years, and also among Far Eastern populations.

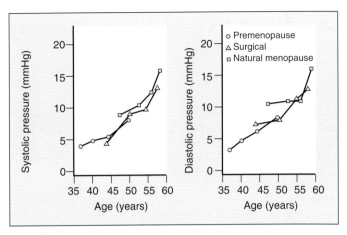

Figure 1.13 The influence of menopause on blood pressure: adjusted blood pressure rise was steeper in postmenopausal women. Reproduced with permission from Staessen J, Bulpitt CJ, Fagard R *et al*. The influence of menopause on blood pressure. *J Hum Hypertens* 1989;**3**:427–33.

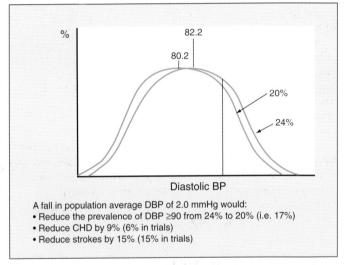

Figure 1.14 The population approach to CVD prevention. Reproduced with permission from Cook NR, Cohen J, Hebert PR *et al*. Implications of small reductions in diastolic blood pressure for primary prevention. *Arch Intern Med* 1995;**155**:701–9.

Further reading

- Clausen J, Jenson G. Blood pressure and mortality: an epidemiological survey with 10 years follow-up. *J Hum Hypertens* 1992;**6**:53–9.
- Collins R, MacMahon S. Blood pressure, antihypertensive drug treatment and the risks of stroke and coronary heart disease. *Br Med Bull* 1994;**50**:272–98.
- Dodson PM, Lip GYH, Eames SM, Gibson JM, Beevers DG. Hypertensive retinopathy: a review of existing classification systems and a suggestion for a simplified grading system. *J Hum Hypertens* 1996;**10**:93–8.
- Stokes J, Kannel WB, Wolf PA, Cupples LA, D'Agostino RB. The relative importance of selective risk factors for various manifestations of cardiovascular disease among men and women from 35 to 64 years. 30 years of follow-up in the Framingham Study. *Circulation* 1987;**75**(Suppl V): V65–V73.
- Whelton PK. Epidemiology of hypertension. *Lancet* 1994;**344**:101–6.

2 Benefits of blood pressure reduction

The last 30 years has seen the introduction of a great many different classes of antihypertensive drugs, the newest agents having relatively few side effects. This means that the millions of hypertensive patients can now have their blood pressure reduced with the minimum reduction in their quality of life, and the benefits of this reduction have been clearly demonstrated. Furthermore, new information has recently become available from the pooled results of all of the randomised controlled trials that have been published in recent years. In addition, we have new information on optimal blood pressure targets during antihypertensive treatment, the treatment of isolated systolic hypertension, the management of hypertensive diabetic patients, and comparisons of the antihypertensive efficacy and tolerability of the different classes of drugs. Further, there are new studies of the role of non-pharmacological measures in the prevention and the treatment of high blood pressure.

Concerns about the safety of the dihydropyridine calcium antagonists have been shown to be unfounded on the basis of large randomised trials, such as SYST-Eur (Systolic-Hypertension-Europe) and HOT (Hypertension Optimal Treatment). Only one long term placebo controlled trial remains to be completed, investigating the role of drug treatment of very elderly patients (the HYVET study).

Thus one could argue that we know who to treat, but more information on *how* to treat is still required, especially with the availability of many different antihypertensive drug classes. Attention is also turning to the management of total cardiovascular risk in hypertensive patients, in particular the role of lipid lowering drugs.

Benefits of BP reduction

- Prevention of myocardial infarction (approximately 20%) and stroke (approximately 40%)
- Decrease target organ damage—reversal of left ventricular hypertrophy and associated complications
- Decrease progression to heart failure or atrial fibrillation
- Improve prothrombotic state

Concerns over treatment of hypertension and trial(s) addressing the question

Concern over adverse effect	Answered by recent trials (examples)
• "J curve"	HOT
• Calcium antagonist crises	SYST-EUR, SYST-CHINA, HOT
• Aspirin use	HOT
• Quality of Life	HOT
• How to treat	ALLHAT, ASCOT
• Lipid lowering therapy	ALLHAT, ASCOT
• New vs old drugs	ALLHAT, ASCOT, LIFE, STOP 2
• Post-stroke	PROGRESS

For abbreviations see page viii

Severe hypertension

Several non-controlled studies were carried out on the treatment of malignant hypertension. The results of treatment were spectacular, with an 80% two-year mortality being transformed with drugs to an 85% five-year survival rate. Clinical trials of severe but non-malignant hypertension were published in the mid 1960s and again the results were impressive, with significant reductions in strokes and heart failure, but a rather disappointing impact on coronary heart disease. The meta-analysis of trials including patients with entry diastolic blood pressure >115 mmHg (severe hypertension) did however clearly show a benefit of treatment on stroke and CHD (Figs 2.1 and 2.2).

Mild to moderate hypertension

Mild hypertension is a symptomless condition and it affects up to 40% of the population. The decision to institute life-long drug treatment must, therefore, be based on clear evidence. It is for this reason that a great many placebo controlled trials have been conducted. Care is needed in their interpretation, however, as clinical trial patients are not typical of patients in general. They tend to be at low overall risk and to be reliable tablet takers. Furthermore, in many studies there was a large fall in blood pressure in patients randomised to placebo or

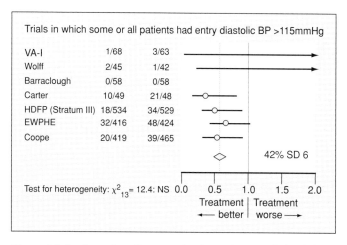

Figure 2.1 Stroke and antihypertensive drugs. Meta-analysis of the trials investigating the benefits of treating hypertension (entry diastolic blood pressure >115 mmHg). For abbreviations see p viii. Reproduced with permission from Collins R, Peto R, MacMahon S *et al.* Blood pressure, stroke, and coronary heart disease. Part 2, short-term reductions in blood pressure: overview of randomised drug trials in their epidemiological context. *Lancet* 1990;**335**:827–38.

inactive therapy. For this reason the results expressed in numbers needed to treat to prevent a stroke or a heart attack seem very large but may be misleading. It is the percentage reduction in cardiovascular events that should be examined and this figure can then be extrapolated to the treatment of patients in more routine clinical practice.

The results of many unconfounded, randomised, controlled trials have been published in the last two to three decades. Some trials addressed the benefits of treating the higher grades of hypertension, five trials were exclusively conducted in older patients, and two concentrated on the benefits of treating isolated systolic hypertension. The four largest trials were the Hypertension Detection and Follow up Programme (HDFP) and the Systolic Hypertension in the Elderly Programme (SHEP) from the USA, and the two Medical Research Council (MRC) trials from Britain which examined separately the treatment of 35- to 64-year-old (MRC 35–64 trial) and 65- to 74-year-old (MRC 65–74 trial) patients respectively.

Each individual trial is open to criticism and several lacked the statistical power to prove that antihypertensive treatment prevents premature deaths. However an overview or meta-analysis of the combined results of the trials provides impressive evidence for the prevention of stroke, heart attack and cardiovascular death rates, with no excess of deaths from other causes (Figs 2.3 and 2.4).

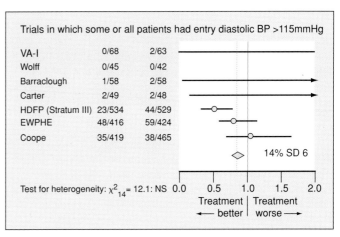

Figure 2.2 Coronary heart disease and antihypertensive drugs. Meta-analysis of the trials investigating the benefits of treating severe hypertension (entry diastolic blood pressure >115 mmHg). Reproduced with permission from Collins R, Peto R, MacMahon S *et al.* Blood pressure, stroke, and coronary heart disease. Part 2, short-term reductions in blood pressure: overview of randomised drug trials in their epidemiological context. *Lancet* 1990;**335**:827–38.

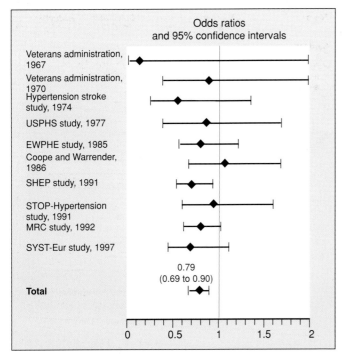

Figure 2.3 Odds ratios and 95% confidence intervals for total (fatal and non-fatal) coronary heart disease related to antihypertensive drug treatment. EWPHE = European Working Party on High Blood Pressure in the Elderly, MRC = Medical Research Council, SHEP = Systolic Hypertension in the Elderly Program, STOP-Hypertension = Swedish Trial in Old Patients with Hypertension, SYST-Eur = Systolic Hypertension in Europe Trial, USPHS = US Public Health Service Hospital Cooperative Study. Reproduced with permission from He J, Whelton PK. Elevated systolic blood pressure as a risk factor for cardiovascular and renal disease. *J Hypertens* 1999;(Suppl 2):S7–S14.

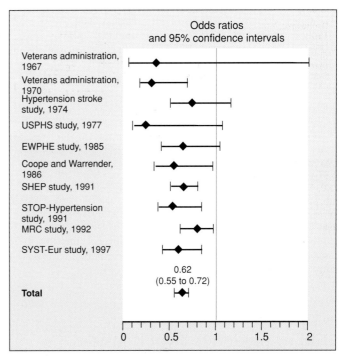

Figure 2.4 Odds ratios and 95% confidence intervals for total (fatal and non-fatal) stroke related to antihypertensive drug treatment. For definitions of trial groups see Figure 2.3. Reproduced with permission from Collins R, Peto R, MacMahon S *et al.* Blood pressure, stroke, and coronary heart disease. Part 2, short-term reductions in blood pressure: overview of randomised drug trials in their epidemiological context. *Lancet* 1990;**335**:827–38.

Preventing strokes

The benefits of reducing blood pressure in preventing strokes were found to be impressive right from the start. The magnitude of the reduction of blood pressure achieved in the trials would be expected to bring about a 35–40% reduction in strokes. The pooled trial data show that the actual reduction achieved was 38% (± 4%). This means that practically all strokes in hypertensive patients that are caused by their hypertension alone should be preventable. These benefits are apparent up to the age of about 80 years and were also seen in patients with isolated systolic hypertension.

Hypertensive patients (particularly the elderly) are at increased risk of dementia due to small vessel disease and even if there is no dementia, there may be some impairment of cognitive function. There is some evidence that lowering blood pressure can lead to some improvement of cognitive function and, indeed, one of the long term outcome trials (SYST-Eur) demonstrated a reduction in the development of dementia.

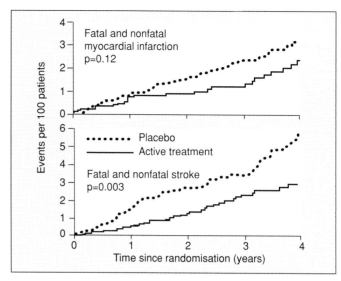

Figure 2.5 The main results of the SYST-Eur trial, comparing placebo (broken line) with the calcium channel blocker, nitrendipine (continuous line) in the treatment of isolated systolic hypertension in the elderly. Reproduced with permission from Staessen JA, Fagard R, Thijs L *et al.* for the SYST-Eur trial investigators. Randomised double blind comparison of placebo and active treatment of older adults with isolated systolic hypertension. *Lancet* 1977;**350**:757–64.

Figure 2.6 Effects of treatment on total and cardiovascular mortality. Data from a meta-analysis of outcome trials – SHEP, SYST-Eur and SYST-China, and subgroups of elderly ISH patients from EWPHE, HEP, STOP, MRC-1, MRC-2. N=15693 pts with ISH. Reproduced with permission from Staessen JA, Gasowski J, Wang *et al.* Risks of untreated and treated isolated systolic hypertension in the elderly: meta-analysis of outcome trials. *Lancet* 2000; **355**: 865–72.

Prevention of heart attacks

The results of the early trials conducted in younger patients had proved a little disappointing in their effects on coronary heart disease; in fact some smaller trials showed no benefits at all although they lacked the statistical power to be certain on this point. However, the pooled data from all of the trials show a somewhat better picture, mainly because of the excellent results in the more recent trials in older patients. Overall the expected reduction in heart attack was 20–25% and the pooled trial data show a 16% (± 4%) reduction, which is highly significant and practically on target. It is interesting to note that much of this reduction was achieved with thiazide diuretic therapy, despite the adverse effects these drugs can have on plasma lipids and glucose tolerance.

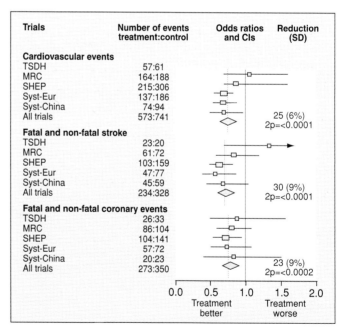

Figure 2.7 Effects of treatment on fatal and non-fatal cardiovascular complications, stroke and coronary events. Data from a meta-analysis of outcome trials – SHEP, SYST-Eur and SYST-China, and subgroups of elderly ISH patients from EWPHE, HEP, STOP, MRC-1, MRC-2. N=15693 pts with ISH. Reproduced with permission from Staessen JA, Gasowski J, Wang *et al.* Risks of untreated and treated isolated systolic hypertension in the elderly: meta-analysis of outcome trials. *Lancet* 2000; **355**: 865–72.

The elderly

Despite clear evidence of the benefits of treating hypertension in patients under 65 years of age, and the strong correlation between raised blood pressure and cardiovascular disease, there has traditionally been some reluctance to treat hypertension in older patients. This is despite the observation that systolic blood pressure rises steadily with increasing age, and the prevalence of hypertension including isolated systolic hypertension (≥ 160/<90 mmHg) is more than 50% in people over the age of 60 years. This originally stemmed from a lack of large clinical trials particularly looking at elderly people and also the view that the rise in blood pressure with age was a normal phenomenon. It was also thought that older people needed their higher pressures to maintain organ perfusion. Thus, treatment might do more harm than good. However, the 1990s saw the publication of several large trials of antihypertensive treatment in elderly patients (Fig 2.8).

All the trials reported a reduction in mortality, which reached significance in the STOP (Swedish Trial of Older Patients) hypertension trial with a fall of 43%. Five of the six trials showed significant reductions in total cardiovascular events and, as might have been expected, this was predominantly the result of a reduction in strokes. In those trials where side effects of drugs and metabolic disturbances were reported, they were all relatively minor. Antihypertensive therapy also reduces the incidence of heart failure by 50% as well as dementia, which are both important conditions in the elderly. The message from these trials is that treatment of hypertension in the patients up to the age of 80 produces a reduction in mortality and morbidity, and regular blood pressure screening should continue up until this age.

The very elderly

Over the age of about 80 years the role of blood pressure in predicting risk becomes more complex because many severely hypertensive patients will have died already. Observational studies tend to show that in the short term people with lower blood pressure have a higher mortality, presumably because their lower pressures are a consequence of existing heart disease or even early cancers. In the long term however this relationship is reversed: the higher the blood pressure the greater the risk of cardiovascular disease, particularly strokes.

With the ageing population, hypertension in the very elderly is becoming an increasing problem, and clearly a long term outcome trial is mandatory. The HYVET study is currently underway comparing a diuretic, with perindopril added where necessary, against placebo in patients aged more than 80 years.

There were some patients aged 80 years or more in the trials in elderly patients, but they were too few to provide reliable information. However the pooled results on treating the very elderly subgroups of patients in these trials does strongly suggest that lowering blood pressure does prevent both fatal and non-fatal strokes (Fig 2.9).

Systolic hypertension

Isolated systolic hypertension (ISH) becomes more common with increasing age. Systolic blood pressure rises sharply with age and this may be the result of thickening of the brachial artery, and may thus reflect arterial damage. Even in the presence of a normal or low diastolic blood pressure, systolic hypertension remains an accurate predictor of cardiovascular

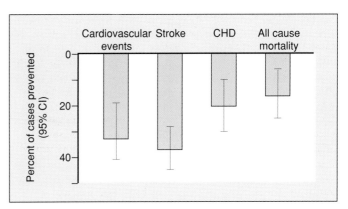

Figure 2.8 Pooled results of the trials of antihypertensive treatment in patients aged over 65 years. Meta-analysis adapted with permission from *Drug treatment of essential hypertension in older people*, Vol. 4, Issue 2, October. NHS Centre for Reviews and Dissemination, 1999.

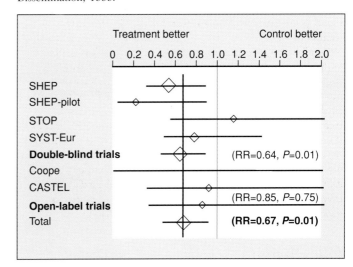

Figure 2.9 Meta-analysis of trials in the very elderly, demonstrating relative risk reduction of stroke of 33%. For definitions of other trial groups see Figure 2.3. Reproduced with permission from Gueyffier F, Bulpitt C, Boissel JP *et al*. Antihypertensive drugs in very old people: a subgroup meta-analysis of randomised controlled trials. INDANA Group. *Lancet* 1999;**353**:793–6.

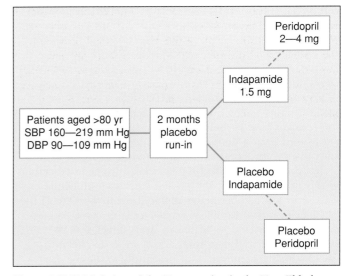

Figure 2.10 Trial design of the Hypertension in the Very Elderly Trial (HYVET). Beckett NS, Connor M, Sadler JD, Fletcher AE on behalf of the HYVET investigators. Orthostatic fall in blood pressure in the very elderly hypertensive. *J Human Hypertens*. 1999;**13**:839–40.

risk. As a consequence, the treatment of isolated systolic hypertension would be expected to reduce cardiovascular risk.

The SHEP study assessed the effect of treating isolated systolic hypertension (systolic blood pressure >160 mmHg with diastolic blood pressure <90 mmHg) in patients of 60 years and over with an average four years and six months follow-up period. The treatment goal was to reduce systolic blood pressure to less than 160 mmHg or by 20 mmHg, whichever was the greater. This study showed a significant reduction in the incidence of stroke and a reduction in all cardiovascular events and mortality. This evidence is supported by subgroup analysis of the patients with ISH from the STOP hypertension trial and the MRC trial in elderly people.

Similarly, the SYST-Eur investigated whether active antihypertensive treatment could reduce cardiovascular complications in elderly patients with isolated systolic hypertension. Patients (>60 years) were randomly assigned to active treatment with the dihydropyridine calcium channel blocker, nitrendipine, with the possible addition of enalapril and hydrochlorothiazide, or matching placebos. In the intention-to-treat analysis, the beween-group difference in blood pressure amounted to 10.1/4.5 mmHg (P<0.001). Active treatment significantly reduced the total incidence of stroke by 42%, all cardiac endpoints by 26%, and all cardiovascular endpoints combined by 31%. Cardiovascular mortality was slightly lower on active treatment (–27%), but all cause mortality was not significantly influenced (–14%). For total and cardiovascular mortality, the benefit of antihypertensive treatment weakened with advancing age and for total mortality it decreased with higher systolic blood pressure at entry. The benefits of active treatment were not independently related to gender or to the presence of cardiovascular complications at entry. Benefits in the reduction of stroke and cardiovascular events were also noted in subgroup analyses of high risk groups, such as those with diabetes (Figure 2.11).

Conclusion

On the basis of a great many randomised placebo controlled trials, we now have reliable information that in all people up to the age of 80 years, if the systolic blood pressure consistently exceeds 160 mmHg, then antihypertensive treatment should be given. The diastolic threshold is less certain but is between 90 and 100 mmHg. Thus the concept of isolated systolic hypertension as a separate entity is incorrect. No matter what the height of the diastolic blood pressure is, the systolic blood pressure is predictive of mortality and morbidity and if raised, it should be reduced. It is also wrong to consider older patients as a separate subgroup, as they are at high risk by virtue of their age and their rising systolic blood pressure, and treatment is very worthwhile.

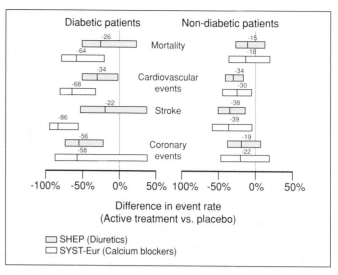

Figure 2.11 Treatment of diabetics with isolated systolic hypertension in the SHEP and SYST-Eur studies. For definitions of trial groups see Figure 2.3. Reproduced with permission from Tuomilehto J, Rastenyte D, Birkenhager WH, *et al.* Effects of calcium-channel blockade in older patients with diabetes and systolic hypertension. SYST-Eur Investigators. *New Engl J Med* 1999;**340**:677–84

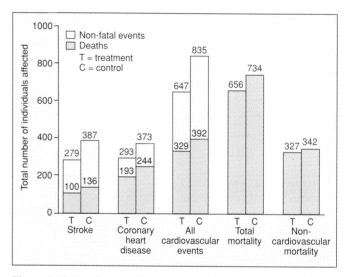

Figure 2.12 Non-fatal and fatal events in older patients with ISH in eight trials of antihypertensive therapy. Data from a meta-analysis of outcome trials – SHEP, SYSTEur and SYST-China, and subgroups of elderly ISH patients from EWPHE, HEP, STOP, MRC-1, MRC-2. N=15693 pts with ISH. Reproduced with permission from Staessen JA, Gasowski J, Wang JG *et al.* Risks of untreated and treated isolated systolic hypertension in the elderly: meta-analysis of outcome trials. *Lancet* 2000; **355**:865–72.

Further reading

- Gueyffier F, Boutitie F, Boissel JP *et al.* Effect of anti-hypertensive drug treatment on cardiovascular outcomes in women and men. A meta-analysis of individual patient data from randomised controlled trials. *Ann Intern Med* 1997;**126**:761–7.
- Swales JD. Pharmacological treatment of hypertension. *Lancet* 1994;**334**:380–5.
- Tuomilehto J, Rastenyte D, Birkenhager WH *et al.* Effects of calcium-channel blockade in older patients with diabetes and systolic hypertension. SYST-Eur Investigators. *New Engl J Med* 1999;**340**:677–84.

3 Epidemiology of hypertension

Hypertension is not an uncommon problem (see Table 3.1). In the Health Survey for England, the prevalence was found to be approximately 50% between the ages of 65 and 74 years, and even higher still above this age. Hypertension is not distributed evenly in the community, and even within the United Kingdom blood pressure varies with geography. For example, a survey of 24 large towns found the lowest mean blood pressure in Shrewsbury, while the highest was in Dunfermline, where the blood pressure was on average 17/11 mmHg higher. On a wider scale differences in blood pressure are even greater, and in some primitive communities hypertension is virtually unknown.

With the increasing age of the general population, the prevalence of hypertension and its complications are likely to increase rather than decrease. In particular, isolated systolic hypertension (systolic BP >160, diastolic BP <90) is particularly common in the elderly. Many will be unaware that they have the condition until they fall victim to its complications of stroke, heart disease, peripheral vascular disease, renal failure, and retinopathy. The detection and treatment of hypertension is therefore vital in the battle to reduce cardiovascular disease and strokes, currently major causes of death in Western countries.

In understanding the problem of hypertension it is important to grasp its impact on the whole population. Within a population blood pressure is a continuous variable (Fig 3.2), distributed in a roughly normal (or Gaussian) manner. Thus there are not two separate groups of individuals (that is, those with and without hypertension), but a continuous range of blood pressures from the lowest to the highest with the majority of individuals falling somewhere in the middle.

This has important implications for public health, as although those with very high blood pressures are individually at very high risk of stroke and coronary heart disease there are very few of them, so even if they all had their hypertension perfectly treated it would have very little impact on the number of strokes and heart attacks occurring in the population as a whole. Conversely the majority of strokes and heart attacks occur in those with only mildly elevated or even "normal" blood pressure. Reducing the blood pressure of the population as a whole by only a few mmHg by public health measures would significantly cut the rate of stroke and coronary heart disease, compared to achieving large reductions in blood pressure in only a few high risk individuals. This should not of course distract us from treating those at highest risk in whom large gains in life expectancy and risk reduction can be made.

Furthermore, the prevalence of hypertension varies depending on the definition used. Using a fairly strict definition of a systolic blood pressure greater than 140 mmHg or a diastolic greater than 90 mmHg or current treatment with antihypertensive medication, the prevalence of hypertension varies from 4% in 18–29 year olds to 65% in the over 80s.

Table 3.1 Estimated prevalence of hypertension pressure (> 160/95) in England and Wales (E&W)

	Age (yr)				
	0–19	20–39	40–59	60–79	80+
Males					
No. E&W	7295 000	7071 000	5596 000	3811 000	386 000
BP ≥ 160/95 (%)	2	7	25	35	50
BP ≥ 160/95 (no.)	146 000	495 000	1399 000	1334 000	193 000
Females					
No. E&W	6925 000	6944 000	5647 000	4939 000	1019 000
BP ≥ 160/95 (%)	1	3	18	37	50
BP ≥ 160/95 (no.)	69 000	208 000	1016 000	1827 000	508 000

Total E&W BP ≥ 160/95 ≃ 7196 000 people

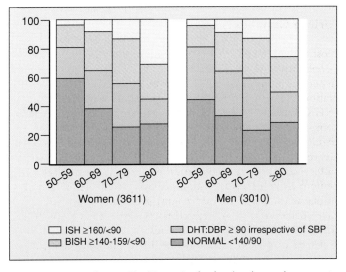

Figure 3.1 Copenhagen City Heart Study showing increasing prevalence of hypertension with age. BISH = borderline isolated systolic hypertension, DHT = diastolic hypertension, ISH = isolated systolic hypertension, NORMAL = normotensives. Adapted from Nielsen WB, Vestbo J, Jensen GB. Isolated systolic hypertension as a major risk factor for stroke and myocardial infarction and an unexploited source of cardiovascular prevention: a prospective population-based study. *J Hum Hypertens* 1995;**9**:175–80.

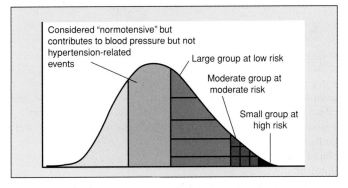

Figure 3.2 Gaussian distribution of blood pressure

Age

In Western societies blood pressure rises with increasing age. However, in rural non-Westernised societies hypertension is rare and the rise in pressure with age is minimal (see Figure 3.3). Migration studies in Africa have, however, shown that members of rural tribes who migrate to urban areas develop a rapid rise in blood pressure within months of arrival. It would seem, therefore, that the rise in blood pressure with age is probably related mainly to socioeconomic and environmental factors.

While systolic blood pressure continues to rise with advancing age, and continues to predict the further development of vascular events, diastolic pressures tend to level off after the age of about 60 years. This may in part explain why diastolic blood pressure is an epidemiologically inferior predictor of risk than systolic pressure. The reason for the flattening out of the diastolic pressure risk at age 60 is uncertain. One explanation is selective mortality, diastolic hypertensives having "died off". Another possibility is a genuine fall in, or a failure to rise of, diastolic pressures in individuals, possibly related to declining cardiac function.

Race

African Caribbeans

Most studies looking at blood pressure in black and white people in Western societies have shown a higher prevalence of hypertension in black people. For example, in the third National Health and Nutrition Examination Survey (NHANES), the prevalence of hypertension in blacks was 32%, compared to 23% in whites. In contrast to these American data, studies in the United Kingdom have produced less clear cut results. For example, Haines *et al.* found no significant difference in average blood pressure levels between black and white men in a North London general practice (134/79 mmHg in blacks compared to 135/78 mmHg in whites); however, more blacks were being treated for hypertension compared to whites (9% vs 5%). In the Northwick Park study, which collected data from 412 white and 141 black individuals, there was a significant difference in mean blood pressure between black and white day shift workers (133/81 mmHg compared to 126/76 mmHg); however, this difference was not noted among night shift workers (139/87 mmHg compared to 135/82 mmHg). The Birmingham Factory study found no significant difference in average blood pressures when comparing black, white and Indo-Asian populations in the west of Birmingham, but there was a small excess in the prevalence of hypertension among blacks.

This is in contrast to the picture in black people living in rural Africa, mentioned above. Even when correction is made for obesity, socioeconomic, and dietary factors, there may still be some racially determined predisposition to hypertension. For example, plasma renin levels are generally lower in black compared with white people; as a result those drugs that antagonise the renin-angiotension system (beta-blockers and angiotensin converting enzyme (ACE) inhibitors) tend to be less effective. Apart from factors related to the renin-angiotensin system and environmental (urbanisation) factors, there may well be factors leading to the higher prevalence of hypertension in blacks, including genetic factors, salt sensitivity, diet (lower potassium intake), and obesity (higher body mass index).

Furthermore, black patients with essential hypertension seem to be at greater risk of developing hypertension related

---

Extremes of age

There is some uncertainty about blood pressure risk and management over age 80–85:

- In the short term, blood pressure is inversely related to risk possibly because pressures have fallen in sicker people with poor health of early pre-clinical cancer.
- In the long term there is a positive correlation between risk and blood pressure.
- Sub-group analysis of patients over the age of 80 years in randomised placebo controlled trials suggests that blood pressure lowering prevents strokes.

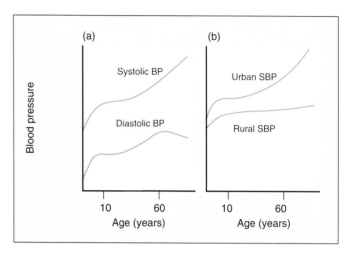

Figure 3.3 Blood pressure and age: (a) normal systolic (upper) and diastolic (lower) pressures; (b) urban societies (upper) and genetically similar tribal communities (lower) in Africa

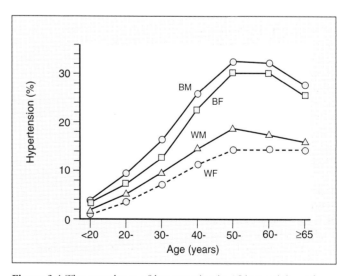

Figure 3.4 The prevalence of hypertension in African-origin and European-origin Americans. BF = black females, BM = black males, WF = white females, WM = white males. Data taken from Stamler J, Stamler R, Riedlinger WF *et al.* Hypertension screening of 1 million Americans. Community Hypertension Evaluation Clinic (CHEC) program, 1973 through 1975. *JAMA* 1976;**235**:2299–306.

cardiovascular complications, particularly strokes and renal failure. This is manifested, in comparison to whites, by a 3-fold increase in overall cardiovascular mortality, a 6-7-fold increase in mortality under the age of 50, the earlier development of hypertensive nephrosclerosis, and a 5-18-fold rise in the incidence of end-stage renal disease, especially in the 25- to 45-year age group. While stroke is commoner in black populations, coronary heart disease is less common than in white populations in the United Kingdom and the Caribbean. However, coronary heart disease has risen sharply in African-Americans.

Other ethnic groups

By contrast, people from the Indian subcontinent, who now live in Western countries, have similar blood pressures to white people, although they have higher rates of coronary heart disease.

Migration studies on Japanese people moving from Japan to the west coast of America have shown that, when they lived in Japan, high blood pressure was common and stroke incidence high, although coronary heart disease was rare. On moving across the Pacific Ocean, there was a reduction in the incidence of hypertension and stroke, but a rise in the incidence of coronary heart disease. These studies strongly suggest that although there are racial differences in the predisposition to hypertension, environmental factors still play a significant role.

Salt

There is now little doubt that salt intake has a direct effect on blood pressure. As stated earlier, migration studies in African and Japanese individuals have shown changes in blood pressure on moving from one environmental background to another, and the factor most likely to be involved in this change in blood pressure was a change in salt intake. The Intersalt project put the salt hypothesis beyond any reasonable doubt. Directly comparable data were obtained from 52 populations in 32 countries, when all the important confounding variables (in particular body mass and alcohol intake) were taken into account. The study showed quite clearly that the rise in blood pressure with advancing age in urban, but not rural, societies resulted from the amount of salt in the diet. This was supported by a recent meta-analysis of the many individual population surveys of blood pressure in relation to salt intake. Furthermore, a larger number of clinical trials have shown a reduction in blood pressure following salt restriction (see Chapter 8).

Potassium

The effect of dietary potassium intake on blood pressure is difficult to separate from that of salt. The Intersalt project did, however, show that high potassium intake was associated with a lower prevalence of hypertension. Studies looking at urinary sodium and potassium ratios in the United States showed marked differences between black and white people, although there was little difference in their sodium intake or excretion. As hypertension is more common in American black people this would support an independent role for potassium in lowering blood pressure. Clinical trials do show that an increase in dietary potassium intake, by eating more fruit, does have a modest antihypertensive effect.

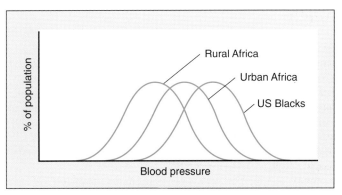

Figure 3.5 Gaussian curves showing blood pressure in populations from rural Africa, urban Africa, and US blacks

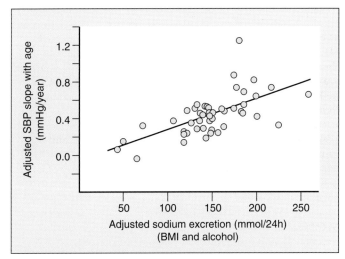

Figure 3.6 Intersalt project: data from 52 centres in 32 countries. Reproduced with permission from Intersalt Cooperative Research Group. *BMJ* 1988;**297**:319–28.

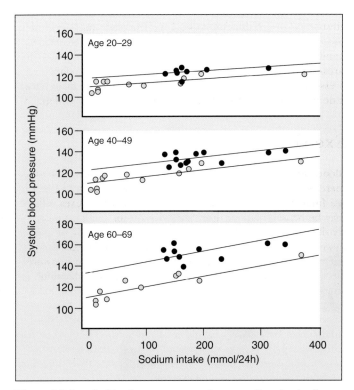

Figure 3.7 Systolic blood pressure according to sodium intake for three age groups in economically developed (●) and undeveloped (○) communities. Reproduced with permission from Law MR, Frost CD, Wald NJ. *BMJ* 1991;**302**:811–15.

Weight

Fat people tend to have higher blood pressures than thin people. Even after taking into account the confounding effects of obese arms and inappropriate cuff sizes on blood pressure measurement, there is still a positive relationship between body mass index (BMI) and blood pressure. Clearly this association is related to an increased caloric intake, although other dietary factors may also be implicated (e.g., obese people may have a higher sodium intake). It has been postulated that obese people can have an increased tendency to exhibit insulin resistance; research is continuing into whether insulin resistance is involved in the pathogenesis of hypertension.

Alcohol

Several epidemiological studies have shown a close positive relationship between alcohol consumption and blood pressure. The Intersalt study also confirmed this trend. Overall, it would appear that the greater the alcohol consumption, the higher the blood pressure, although teetotallers appear to have slightly higher blood pressures than moderate drinkers. The reversibility of alcohol related hypertension has also been shown in population surveys, and in alcohol loading and restriction studies. The mechanisms of the alcohol/blood pressure relationship are uncertain but they are not explained by body mass index or salt intake.

Stress

It has been suggested that psychological or environmental stress may play a part in the aetiology of hypertension. There is, however, little reliable evidence to support this. Studies of environmental stress levels in relation to hypertension have frequently been confounded by other environmental or lifestyle factors. Although stressful stimuli may cause an acute rise in blood pressure, it is still doubtful whether this has any significance in the long term. A reduction in psychological stress through biofeedback techniques may reduce blood pressure in the clinic; however, these techniques seem to have little effect on ambulatory home blood pressure recordings.

Exercise

Blood pressure rises sharply during physical activity, although there is evidence that people who undertake regular exercise are fitter and healthier and have lower blood pressures. This may be because such people have a healthier diet and more sensible drinking and smoking habits. A recent study has, however, shown that there is an independent relationship between increased levels of exercise and lower blood pressures. The study suggests that vigorous exercise might be harmful, but all other grades of exercise are beneficial.

Table 3.2 The prevalence of hypertension in relation to body weight. Data taken from Stamler J *et al. JAMA* 1976;**235**: 2299–306.

	Percent hypertensive	
	20–39 yr	*40–69 yr*
Weight		
Underweight	4.6	19.0
Normal	6.2	24.1
Overweight	14.9	37.1

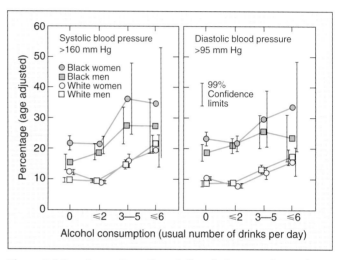

Figure 3.8 Prevalence of systolic and diastolic hypertension. Kaiser Permanent Health Examination Program (USA). Reproduced with permission from Klatsky AL, Friedman GD, Siegelaub AB, Gerard MJ. *New Engl J Med* 1977;**296**:1194–200.

While there is good evidence that acute stressful stimuli do raise blood pressure, there is little convincing evidence that chronic stress causes hypertension

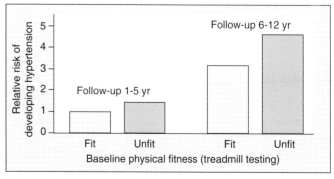

Figure 3.9 Physical fitness and the development of hypertension. Reproduced with permission from Blair SN, Goodyear NN, Gibbons LW, Cooper KH. Physical fitness and incidence of hypertension in healthy normotensive men and women. *JAMA* 1984;**252**:487–90.

Further reading

- Dustan HP. Mechanisms of hypertension associated with obesity. *Ann Intern Med* 1983;**98**:860–4.
- Elliot P, Stamler J, Nichols R *et al*. Intersalt revisited: further analysis of 24 hr sodium excretion and blood pressure within and across populations. *BMJ* 1996;**312**:1249–53.
- Grim CE, Luft FC, Millar JZ *et al*. Racial differences in blood pressure in Evans County, Georgia: relationship to sodium and potassium intake and plasma renin activity. *J Chronic Dis* 1980;**33**:87–94.
- Rose G. Sick individuals and sick populations. *Int J Epidemiol* 1985;**14**:32–8.
- Shaper AG, Wannamethee G, Whincup PH. Alcohol and blood pressure in middle aged British men. *J Hum Hypertens* 1988;**2**:71–8.
- Staessen J, Fagard R, Amery A. The relationship between body weight and blood pressure. *J Hum Hypertens* 1988;**2**:201–7.

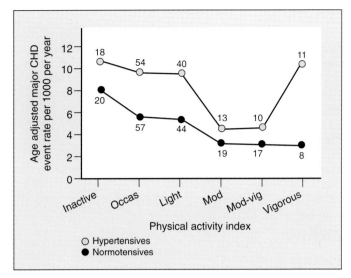

Figure 3.10 Exercise and coronary heart disease. Reproduced with permission from Wannamethee G, Walker M. Physical activity, hypertension and risk of heart attack in men without evidence of ischemic heart disease. *J Hum Hypertens* 1994;**8**:3–10.

4   The pathophysiology of hypertension

There is still much uncertainty about the pathophysiology of hypertension. A small number of patients (between 2% and 5%) have an underlying renal or adrenal disease as the cause for their raised blood pressure. In the remainder, however, no clear single identifiable cause is found and their condition is labelled "essential hypertension". A number of physiological mechanisms are involved in the maintenance of normal blood pressure and their derangement may play a part in the development of essential hypertension.

It is probable that a great many interrelated factors contribute to the raised blood pressure in hypertensive patients and their relative roles may differ between individuals. Among the factors that have been intensively studied are salt intake, obesity and insulin resistance, the renin-angiotensin system, and the sympathetic nervous system. In the past few years, a number of other factors have been evaluated, including genetics, endothelial dysfunction (as manifested by changes in endothelin and nitric oxide), low birth weight and intrauterine nutrition, as well as neurovascular anomalies.

Cardiac output and peripheral resistance

Maintenance of a normal blood pressure is dependent on the balance between the cardiac output and peripheral vascular resistance. Most patients with essential hypertension have a normal cardiac output but a raised peripheral resistance. Peripheral resistance is determined not by large arteries or the capillaries but by small arterioles, the walls of which contain smooth muscle cells. Contraction of smooth muscle cells is thought to be related to a rise in intracellular calcium concentration, which may explain the vasodilatory effect of drugs that block the calcium channels. Prolonged smooth muscle constriction is thought to induce structural changes with thickening of the arteriolar vessel walls possibly mediated by angiotensin, leading to an irreversible rise in peripheral resistance.

It has been postulated that in very early hypertension the peripheral resistance is not raised and the elevation of the blood pressure is caused by a raised cardiac output, which is related to sympathetic overactivity. The subsequent rise in peripheral arteriolar resistance might therefore develop in a compensatory manner to prevent the raised pressure being transmitted to the capillary bed where it would substantially affect cell homeostasis.

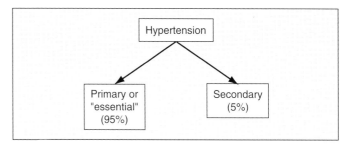

Figure 4.1 The relative frequency of primary and secondary hypertension

Physiological mechanisms involved in development of essential hypertension

Cardiac output
Peripheral resistance
Renin–angiotensin–alsosterone system
Autonomic nervous system
Other factors
   Bradykinin
   Endothelin
   EDRF (endothelial derived relaxing factor) or nitric oxide (NO)
   ANP (atrial natriuretic peptide).
   Ouabain

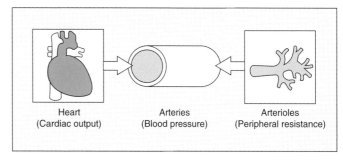

Figure 4.2 The heart, arteries and arterioles in hypertension

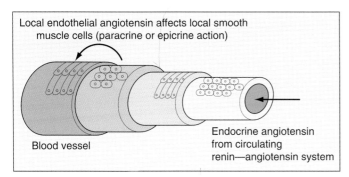

Figure 4.3 Local vs systemic renin-angiotensin systems

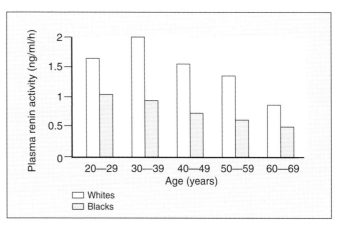

Figure 4.4 Plasma renin in black and white hypertensives. From Freis ED, Materson BJ, Flamenbaum V. Comparison of propranolol or hydrochlorothiazide alone for treatment of hypertension: III evaluation of the renin–angiotensin system. *Am J Med* 1983;**74**:1029–41.

Renin-angiotensin system

The renin-angiotensin system may be the most important of the endocrine systems that affect the control of blood pressure. Renin is secreted from the juxtaglomerular apparatus of the kidney in response to glomerular underperfusion or a reduced salt intake. It is also released in response to stimulation from the sympathetic nervous system. Renin is responsible for converting renin substrate (angiotensinogen) to angiotensin I, a physiologically inactive substance which is rapidly converted to angiotensin II in the lungs by angiotensin converting enzyme (ACE). Angiotensin II is a potent vasoconstrictor and thus causes a rise in blood pressure. In addition it stimulates the release of aldosterone from the zona glomerulosa of the adrenal gland, which results in a further rise in blood pressure related to sodium and water retention. The circulating renin-angiotensin system is not thought to be directly responsible for the rise in blood pressure in essential hypertension. In particular, many hypertensive patients have low levels of renin and angiotensin II (especially the elderly and black people), and drugs that block the renin-angiotensin system are not particularly effective. There is, however, increasing evidence that there are important non-circulating "local" renin-angiotensin epicrine or paracrine systems, which also control blood pressure. Local renin systems have been reported in the kidney, the heart and the arterial tree. They may have important roles in regulating regional blood flow.

Autonomic nervous system

Sympathetic nervous system stimulation can cause both arteriolar constriction and arteriolar dilatation. Thus the autonomic nervous system has an important role in maintaining a normal blood pressure. It is also important in the mediation of short term changes in blood pressure in response to stress and physical exercise. There is, however, little evidence to suggest that epinephrine (adrenaline) and norepinephrine (noradrenaline) have any clear role in the aetiology of hypertension. Nevertheless, their effects are important, not least because drugs that block the sympathetic nervous system do lower blood pressure and have a well established therapeutic role. It is probable that hypertension is related to an interaction between the autonomic nervous system and the renin-angiotensin system, together with other factors, including sodium, circulating volume, and some of the more recently described hormones, see Figure 4.7.

- Cross transplantation experiments with kidneys of hypertensive rats transferred to normotensives, and vice versa, strongly suggest that hypertension has its origins in the kidneys.
- Similarly human evidence from renal transplant recipients shows that they are more likely to develop hypertension if the donors' relatives are hypertensive.
- This essential hypertension may be due to a genetically inherited abnormality of sodium handling.

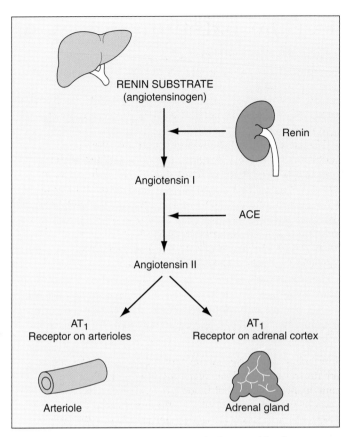

Figure 4.5 Renin-angiotensin system and effects on blood pressure and aldosterone release

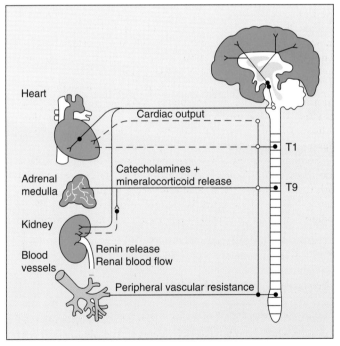

Figure 4.6 The autonomic nervous system and its control of blood pressure. Reproduced with permission from Swales JD, Sever PS, Plart WS. *Clinical atlas of hypertension*. London and New York: Gower Medical Publishing, 1991.

Endothelial dysfunction

Vascular endothelial cells play a key role in cardiovascular regulation by producing a number of potent local vasoactive agents, including the vasodilator molecule nitric oxide (NO) and the vasoconstrictor peptide endothelin (ET-1). Dysfunction of the endothelium has been implicated in human essential hypertension.

Modulation of endothelial function is an attractive therapeutic option in attempting to minimise some of the important complications of hypertension. Clinically effective antihypertensive therapy appears to restore impaired production of nitric oxide, but does not seem to restore the impaired endothelium dependent vascular relaxation or vascular response to endothelial agonists. This indicates that such endothelial dysfunction is primary and becomes irreversible once the hypertensive process has become established.

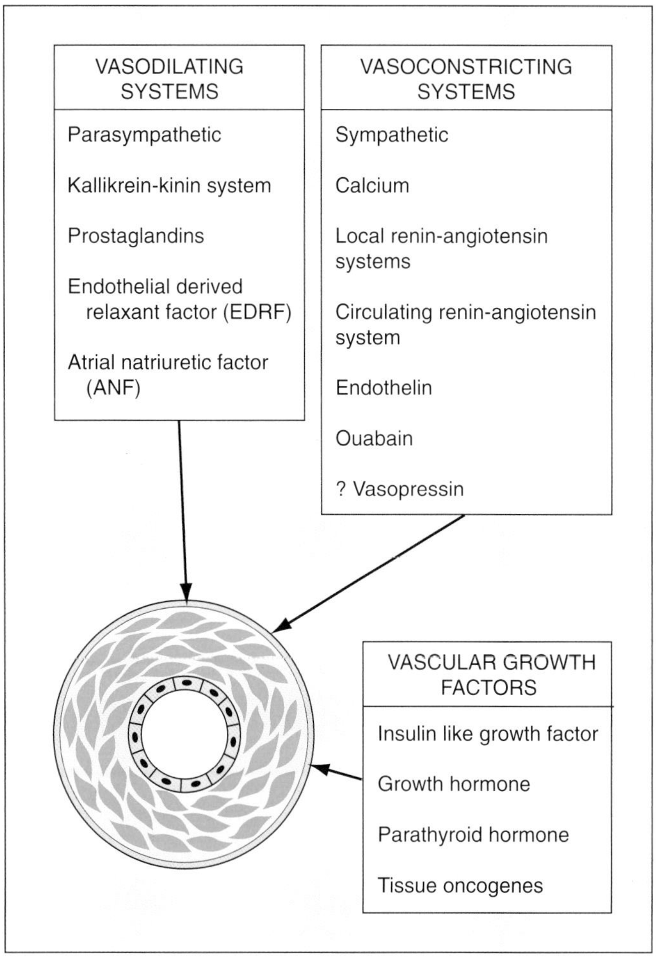

Vasoactive substances

Many other vasoactive systems and mechanisms affecting sodium transport and vascular tone are involved in the maintenance of a normal blood pressure. It is not clear, however, what part these play in the development of essential hypertension. Bradykinin is a potent vasodilator that is inactivated by angiotensin converting enzyme. Consequently, the ACE inhibitors may exert some of their effect by blocking bradykinin inactivation.

Endothelin is a recently discovered, powerful, vascular, endothelial vasoconstrictor, which may produce a salt sensitive rise in blood pressure. It also activates local renin-angiotensin systems. Endothelial derived relaxant factor (EDRF), now known to be nitric oxide (NO), is produced by arterial and venous endothelium and diffuses through the vessel wall into the smooth muscle causing vasodilatation.

Atrial natriuretic peptide (ANP) is a hormone secreted from atria of the heart in response to increased blood volume. Its effect is to increase sodium and water excretion from the kidney as a sort of natural diuretic. A defect in this system may cause fluid retention and hypertension.

Sodium transport across vascular smooth muscle cell walls is also thought to influence blood pressure via its interrelationship with calcium transport. Ouabain may be a naturally occurring steroid-like substance which is thought to interfere with cell sodium and calcium transport, giving rise to vasoconstriction.

Figure 4.7 The control of peripheral arteriolar resistance. Reproduced with permission from Beevers DG, MacGregor GA. *Hypertension in Practice*, third edition. London: Martin Dunitz, 1999.

The thrombotic paradox of hypertension (The Birmingham Paradox)

While the blood vessels are exposed to high pressures in hypertension, the main complications of hypertension (stroke and myocardial infarction) paradoxically are thrombotic rather than haemorrhagic.

Hypercoagulability

Patients with hypertension demonstrate abnormalities of vessel wall (endothelial dysfunction or damage), the blood constituents (abnormal levels of haemostatic factors, platelet activation, and fibrinolysis), and blood flow (rheology, viscosity, and flow reserve), suggesting that hypertension confers a prothrombotic or hypercoagulable state. These components appear to be related to target organ damage, long term prognosis and some may be altered by antihypertensive treatment.

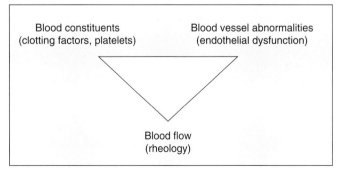

Figure 4.8 Virchow's triad and the prothrombotic state in hypertension

Insulin sensitivity

Epidemiologically there is a clustering of several risk factors including obesity, hypertension, glucose intolerance, diabetes mellitus, and hyperlipidaemia. This has led to the suggestion that these represent a single syndrome (metabolic syndrome X or Reaven's syndrome), with a final common pathway to cause raised blood pressure and vascular damage. Indeed some hypertensive patients who are not obese display resistance to insulin. There are many objections to this hypothesis, but it may explain why the hazards of cardiovascular risk are synergistic or multiplicative rather than just additive.

Genetic factors

Although separate genes and genetic factors have been linked to the development of essential hypertension, multiple genes are most likely contribute to the development of the disorder in a particular individual. It is therefore extremely difficult to accurately determine the relative contributions of each of these genes. Nevertheless, hypertension is about twice as common in subjects who have one or two hypertensive parents, and many epidemiological studies suggest that genetic factors account for approximately 30% of the variation in blood pressure in various populations. This figure can be derived from comparisons of parents with their monozygotic and dizygotic twin children as well as their other children and with adopted children. Some familial concordance is however due to shared lifestyle (chiefly dietary) factors.

Some specific genetic mutations can rarely cause hypertension. Experimental models of genetic hypertension have shown that the inherited tendency to hypertension resides primarily in the kidney. For example, animal and human studies show that a transplanted kidney from a hypertensive donor raises the blood pressure and increases antihypertensive drug requirements in recipients coming from "normotensive" families. Conversely a kidney from a normotensive donor does not raise the blood pressure in the recipient.

Increased plasma levels of angiotensinogen, the protein substrate acted upon by renin to generate angiotensin I, have also been reported in hypertensive subjects and in children of hypertensive parents.

Hypertension is rarely found in rural or "tribal" areas of Africa, but it is very common in African cities and in black populations in Britain and the United States. While the rural/urban differences in Africa are clearly due to lifestyle and dietary factors, the finding that hypertension is commoner in blacks compared with whites may have some genetic basis. There is some evidence from salt loading studies in medical students that US blacks are more susceptible to a given salt load than whites, and may be more sensitive to the beneficial effects of salt restriction.

Intrauterine influences

There is increasing evidence that fetal influences, particularly birth weight, may be a determinant of blood pressure in adult life. For example, babies who are small at birth are more likely to have higher blood pressures during adolescence and to be hypertensive as adults. Small-for-age babies are also more likely to have metabolic abnormalities that have been associated with the later development of hypertension and cardiovascular disease, such as insulin resistance, diabetes

Examples of specific genetic mutations causing hypertension

- Liddles syndrome, a disorder associated with hypertension, low plasma renin and aldosterone levels, and hypokalaemia, all of which respond to amiloride, an inhibitor of the distal renal epithelial sodium channel
- Glucocorticoid-remediable aldosteronism (GRA), a disorder mimicking Conn's syndrome in which there is a chimeric gene formed from portions of the 11β-hydroxylase gene and the aldosterone synthase gene. This defect results in hyperaldosteronism, which is responsive to dexamethasone and has a high incidence of stroke
- Congenital adrenal hyperplasia due to 11β-hydroxylase deficiency, a disorder that has been associated with 10 different mutations of the *CYP11B1* gene
- Syndrome of apparent mineralocorticoid excess (AME), arising from mutations in the gene encoding the kidney enzyme 11α-hydroxysteroid dehydrogenase; the defective enzyme allows normal circulating concentrations of cortisol (which are much higher than those of aldosterone) to activate the mineralocorticoid receptors
- Congenital adrenal hyperplasia due to 17α-hydroxylase deficiency, a disorder with hyporeninaemia hypoaldosteronism, absent secondary sexual characteristics and hypokalaemia
- Gordon's syndrome (pseudo-hypoaldosteronism): familial hypertension with hyperkalaemia, possibly related to the long arm of chromosome 17
- Sporadic case reports of familial inheritance of phaeochromocytoma (Multiple Endocrine Neoplasia, MEN-II syndrome), Cushing's syndrome, Conn's syndrome, renal artery stenosis due to fibromuscular dysplasia

Other associations
- Angiotensinogen gene may be related to hypertension
- Angiotensin converting enzyme (ACE) gene may be related to left ventricular hypertrophy or hypertensive nephropathy
- α-Adducin gene may be related to salt sensitive hypertension

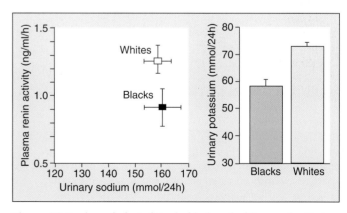

Figure 4.9 Renin and electrolytes in black and white people. He J, Klag MJ, Appel LJ, Charleston J, Whelton PK. The renin–angiotensin system and blood pressure; differences between blacks and whites. *Am J Hypertens* 1999;**12**:555–62.

mellitus, hyperlipidaemia, and abdominal obesity ("the Barker hypothesis"). Insulin resistance almost certainly contributes to the increased prevalence of coronary disease seen in adults of low birth weight.

It is possible however that genetic factors influence the Barker hypothesis. Mothers with above average blood pressure in pregnancy give birth to smaller babies who subsequently develop above average blood pressure themselves and eventually hypertension. It is entirely likely that the similarity of blood pressures in mother and child are genetic and, in a modern "healthy" society, unrelated to intrauterine undernutrition.

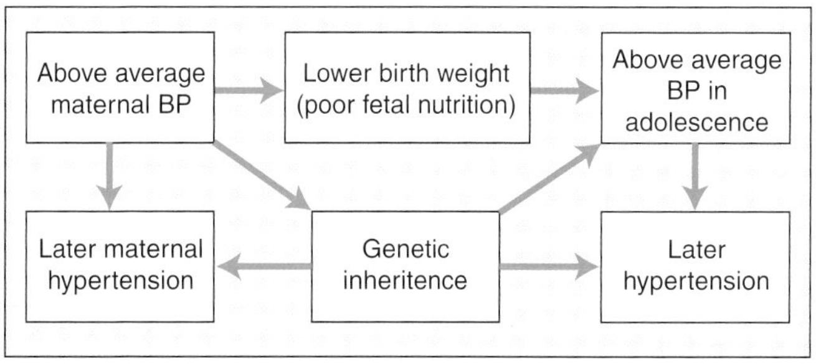

Figure 4.10 Possible mechanisms to explain why low birth weight babies are more likely to develop hypertension in later life

Diastolic dysfunction

In hypertensive left ventricular hypertrophy (LVH), the ventricle cannot relax normally in diastole. Thus, to produce the necessary increase in ventricular input especially during exercise, there is an increase in left atrial pressure rather than the normal reduction in ventricular pressure, which produces a suction effect as described above. This can lead to an elevation in pulmonary capillary pressure that is sufficient to induce pulmonary congestion. The rise in atrial pressure can also lead to atrial fibrillation, and in hypertrophied ventricles dependent on atrial systole, the loss of atrial transport can result in a significant reduction in stroke volume and pulmonary oedema. Exercise induced subendocardial ischaemia can also produce an "exaggerated" impairment of diastolic relaxation of the hypertrophied myocardium.

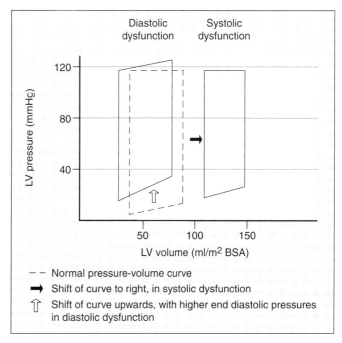

Figure 4.11 Pressure-volume curves demonstrating diastolic/systolic dysfunction

Further reading

- Barker DJP, Osmond C, Golding J, Kuh D, Wadsworth MEJ. Growth in utero, blood pressure in childhood and adult life and mortality from cardiovascular disease. *BMJ* 1989;**298**:564–7.
- Dzau VJ. Circulating versus local renin–angiotensin system in cardiovascular homeostasis. *Circulation* 1988;**77**(Suppl 1): 1-4–1-13.
- Harrap SB. Hypertension: genes versus environment. *Lancet* 1994;**344**:169–71.
- Hughes AD, Schachter M. Hypertension and blood vessels. *Br Med Bull* 1994;**50**:356–70.
- Kurtz TW. Genetic models of hypertension. *Lancet* 1994;**344**:167–8.
- Lip GYH, Li-Saw-Hee FL. Does hypertension confer a hypercoagulable state? *J Hypertens* 1998;**16**:913–16.
- Mathias CJ. Role of sympathetic efferent nerves in blood pressure regulation and in hypertension. *Hypertension* 1991;**18**:22–30.
- Sagnella G, Macgregor GA. Atrial natriuretic peptides. *Q J Med* 1990;**77**:1001–7.

5 Blood pressure measurement

Part I Sphygmomanometry: factors common to all techniques

History and background

Sphygmomanometry has evolved over nearly three centuries, but conventional sphygmomanometry, the technique with which we are all so familiar in clinical practice, was introduced just over a century ago by Riva-Rocci in 1896 and modified by Korotkoff in 1905. Indeed, when sphygmomanometry was first introduced to clinical practice, it was regarded as so innovative as to have little future; one commentator, writing in 1895, while acknowledging that "the middle-aged and successful physician may slowly and imperceptibly lose the exquisite sensitiveness of his finger tips through repeated attacks of gouty neuritis", doubted if the sphygmomanometer would be welcomed by "the overworked and underpaid general practitioner, already loaded with thermometer, stethoscope, etc., etc.,...". And yet the technique has lived on for over a century, earning the reputation of having contributed more to cardiovascular science than any other measurement technique in clinical medicine.[1]

Blood pressure measurement is one of the few scientific measurements undertaken by doctors in the course of clinical assessment and it occupies more of the nurse's time, both on the wards, in the accident and emergency department and in the outpatients departments, than any other measurement. The situation is similar in family practice. The consequences of decisions arising from the measurement of blood pressure may be crucial to patient management both in the short term and, perhaps more importantly, the level of blood pressure recorded may influence the quality of existence for the remainder of a patient's life.

The mercury sphygmomanometer, which has served us so well for so long, is now being relegated to the museum shelves and a new era in blood pressure measurement is dawning. The reasons for this are threefold. Firstly, the pressure from environmentalists to ban mercury as a toxic substance is likely to be persuasive, as indeed it has been in Scandinavian countries. Secondly, accurate automated devices will soon

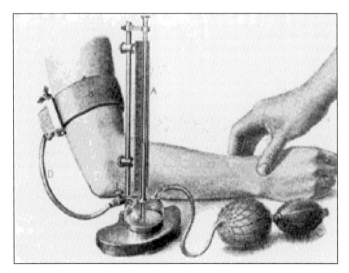

Figure 5.1 Riva-Rocci sphygmomanometer. Reproduced with permission from O'Brien E, Fitzgerald D. The history of indirect blood pressure measurement. In: *Blood pressure measurement*. O'Brien E, O'Malley K, eds. Amsterdam: Elsevier, 1991:1–54.

Historical milestones in blood pressure measurement
• 1733: The Reverend Stephen Hales performed his famous experiment demonstrating that blood rose to a height of 8 feet 3 inches in a glass tube placed in the artery of a horse
• 1828: Blood pressure in animals measured directly with a mercury sphygmomanometer by Jean-Leonard Marie Poiseuille
• 1847: Introduction of the kymograph by Carl Ludwig
• 1855: Introduction of the sphygmograph by Karl Vierordt
• 1850–90: Development of sphygmographs by Marey, Mahomed and Dudgeon
• 1880: Introduction of the "Sphygmomanometer" of von Basch
• 1880–90: Modifications to von Basch sphygmomanometer by Potain, Hill and Barnard
• 1896: Scipione Riva-Rocci introduced an arm-occluding mercury sphygmomanometer which could record systolic blood pressure accurately in clinical conditions
• 1897: Hill and Barnard developed an arm-occluding aneroid sphygmomanometer
• 1905: The Russian surgeon, Nicolai Sergeivich Korotkov, presented the technique of auscultatory measurement of systolic and diastolic blood pressure to the Imperial Military Academy in St. Petersburg
• 1904: Theodore Janeway drew attention to the variability of blood pressure and the striking response to stresses, such as surgery, tobacco and anxiety
• 1940: Ayman and Goldshine showed that blood pressure measured at home was lower than in the clinic
• 1944: Smirk assessed blood pressure behaviour in the individual by measuring basal blood pressure
• 1964: George Pickering showed for the first time how constant and profound was the fall in blood pressure recorded during sleep
• 1964: Hinman described the first truly portable ambulatory system for the non-invasive measurement of blood pressure—the Remler
• 1992: Ambulatory blood pressure measurement passes from research to clinical practice
• 1991: Normal levels for ambulatory blood pressure described
• 1997: Ambulatory blood pressure measurement shown to result in less drug treatment than conventional measurement
• 1998: Ambulatory blood pressure shown to be a better predictor of prognosis than conventional measurement

replace the conventional technique, which for all that we may owe it, is flawed by inaccuracy due to observer prejudice. Third, the development of computer assisted techniques for blood pressure measurement, by allowing examination of blood pressure measurements taken over periods of time, has demonstrated how misleading single measurements may be in assessing blood pressure. The availability of techniques for measuring ambulatory blood pressure has shown that blood pressure is influenced by a number of factors, which include activity, sleep, and anxiety. So attention has turned from the casual blood pressure measurement, often obtained under unusual circumstances, to profiles of blood pressure behaviour. This trend has been hastened by the realisation that ambulatory blood pressures are more accurate predictors of cardiovascular outcome than the conventional technique of measurement.[1]

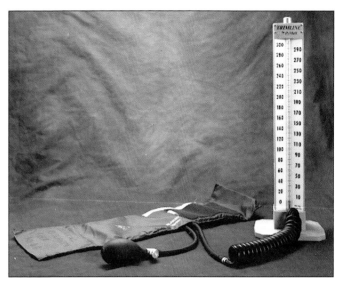

Figure 5.2 Mercury sphygmomanometer

Methods of blood pressure measurement

Most devices for measuring blood pressure are dependent on one common feature, namely, occluding the artery of an extremity (arm, wrist, finger, or leg) with an inflatable cuff to measure blood pressure either oscillometrically, or by detection of Korotkoff sounds. Other techniques, which are not dependent on limb occlusion, such as pulse-waveform analysis, can also be used, but these have little application in clinical practice. The array of techniques available today owe their origins to the conventional technique of auscultatory blood pressure measurement, and these new techniques must indeed be shown to be as accurate as the traditional mercury sphygmomanometer. Since the introduction of sphygmomanometry, mercury and aneroid sphygmomanometers have been the most popular devices for measuring blood pressures.

Important factors affecting measurement

- The inherent variability of blood pressure
- The defence reaction
- The limitations of the device being used
- The accuracy of the device
- Blood pressure is not as easily measured in some groups, such as elderly people

---

Factors affecting blood pressure measurement

No matter which device is used to measure blood pressure, it must be recognised that blood pressure is a variable haemodynamic phenomenon, which is influenced by many factors, not least being the circumstances of measurement itself. These influences on blood pressure can be significant, often accounting for rises in systolic blood pressure greater than 20 mmHg, and if they are ignored, or unrecognised, hypertension will be diagnosed erroneously and inappropriate management instituted. These factors have to be carefully considered in all circumstances of blood pressure measurement – self measurement by patients, conventional measurement, measurement with automated devices whether in a doctor's surgery, an ambulance, a pharmacy, or in hospital using sophisticated technology.[2,3]

Variability of blood pressure

The observer must be aware of the considerable variability that may occur in blood pressure from moment to moment with respiration, emotion, exercise, meals, tobacco, alcohol, temperature, bladder distension, and pain, and that blood pressure is also influenced by age, race, and circadian variation. It is usually at its lowest during sleep. It is not always possible to modify these many factors but we can

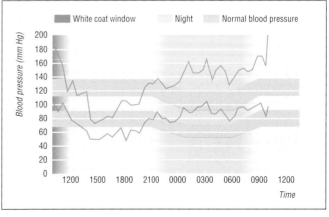

Figure 5.3 Example of a normal ambulatory blood pressure pattern plotted by the DABL® Program showing a marked variability of blood pressure.

minimise their effect by taking them into account in reaching a decision as to the relevance or otherwise of a particular blood pressure measurement.[2]

Insofar as is practical the patient should be relaxed in a quiet room at a comfortable temperature and a short period of rest should precede the measurement. When it is not possible to achieve optimum conditions, this should be noted with the blood pressure reading – for example, "BP 154/92, R arm, V phase (patient very nervous)".

"White coat" hypertension

Anxiety raises blood pressure, often by as much as 30 mmHg. This may be regarded as a physiological reaction, often referred to as the "fight and flight" phenomenon, or "defence" or "alarm" reaction. It is commonly seen in the accident and emergency departments of hospitals when patients are frightened and extremely anxious, but it may also occur in family doctors' surgeries and in the outpatients department. It may occur in normotensive and hypertensive subjects. The degree of this reaction varies greatly from patient to patient being absent in many, and it is usually reduced or abolished altogether with reassurance and familiarisation with the technique and circumstances of blood pressure measurement. Its importance in practice is that decisions to lower blood pressure, and especially to administer drugs, should never be made on the basis of measurements taken in circumstances where the defence reaction is likely to be present.

White coat hypertension is a condition in which a normotensive subject becomes hypertensive during blood pressure measurement, but pressures then settle to normal outside the medical environment. It is best demonstrated by ambulatory blood pressure measurement (ABPM).

No one group seems to be exempt from the white coat phenomenon; it may affect the young, the elderly, normotensive and hypertensive subjects, and pregnant women. In young subjects with borderline elevation of conventional blood pressure, identification of white coat hypertension can be of considerable importance in avoiding undue penalties for insurance and employment. Moreover, there are no characteristics that allow for the identification of the phenomenon, other than by obtaining blood pressures away from the medical environment, either by self measurement in the home or with ABPM, which is the technique of choice. Patients diagnosed as "hypertensive" with conventional measurement in whom white coat hypertension is considered a possibility should have ABPM performed before they are labelled "hypertensive", and certainly before treatment is instigated.

Posture of subject

Posture affects blood pressure, with a general tendency for it to increase from the lying to the sitting or standing position. However, in most people posture is unlikely to lead to significant error in blood pressure measurement provided the arm is supported at heart level. None the less, it is advisable to standardise posture for individual patients and in practice blood pressure is usually measured in the sitting position. Patients should be comfortable whatever their position. No information is available on the optimal time that a subject should remain in a particular position before a measurement, but three minutes is suggested for the lying and sitting

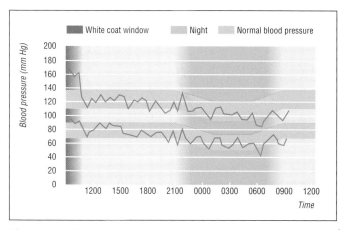

Figure 5.4 White coat hypertension

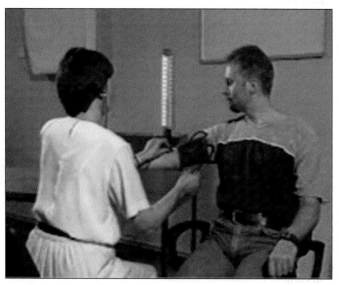

Figure 5.5 Patient in standard seated position.

positions and one minute standing. Some antihypertensive drugs cause postural hypotension, and when this is expected blood pressure should be measured both lying and standing.[2]

Arm support

If the arm in which measurement is being made is unsupported, as tends to happen if the subject is sitting or standing, isometric exercise is performed raising blood pressure and heart rate. Diastolic blood pressure may be raised by as much as 10% by having the arm extended and unsupported during blood pressure measurement. The effect of isometric exercise is greater in hypertensive patients and in those taking beta-blockers. It is essential, therefore that the arm is supported during blood pressure measurement and this is best achieved in practice by having the observer hold the subject's arm at the elbow, although in research the use of an arm support on a stand has much to commend it.[2]

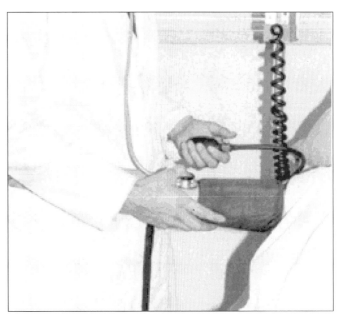

Figure 5.6 Arm support in standing position

Arm position

The arm must also be horizontal at the level of the heart as denoted by the midsternal level. Dependency of the arm below heart level leads to an overestimation of systolic and diastolic pressures and raising the arm above heart level leads to underestimation. The magnitude of this error can be as great as 10 mmHg for systolic and diastolic pressures. This source of error becomes especially important in the sitting and standing positions, when the arm is likely to be dependent by the subject's side. However, it has been demonstrated that even in the supine position an error of 5 mmHg for diastolic pressure may occur if the arm is not supported at heart level.[2,3] Arm position has become an important issue for self measurement of blood pressure with the manufacture of devices for measuring blood pressure at the wrist, which are proving very popular because of the ease of measurement. Many of these devices are inherently inaccurate, but measurement is extremely inaccurate if the wrist is not held at heart level during measurement.

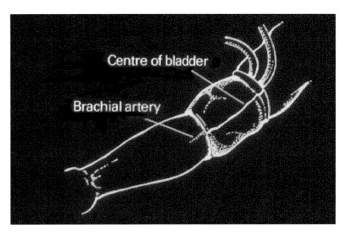

Figure 5.7 Placement of cuff

Which arm

This topic remains controversial as some studies, but not all, using simultaneous measurement have demonstrated significant differences between arms.[2] However, the fact that blood pressure differences between arms are variable makes the issue even more problematical. A reasonable policy is to measure blood pressure in both arms at the initial examination, and if differences greater than 20 mmHg for systolic or 10 mmHg for diastolic pressure are present on three consecutive readings the patient should be referred to a cardiovascular centre for further evaluation.

The cuff and bladder

The cuff is an inelastic cloth that encircles the arm and encloses the inflatable rubber bladder. It is secured around the arm most commonly by means of Velcro on the adjoining surfaces of the cuff, occasionally by wrapping a tapering end into the encircling cuff, and rarely by hooks. Velcro surfaces must be effective, and when they lose their grip the cuff should be discarded. It should be possible to remove the bladder from the cuff so that the latter can be washed from time to time.[2]

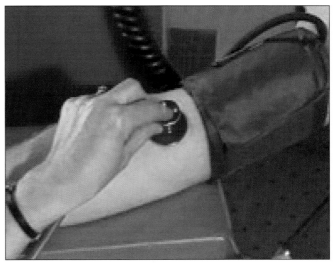

Figure 5.8 Placement of stethoscope

"Cuff hypertension"

However sophisticated a blood pressure measuring device may be, if it is dependent on cuff occlusion of the arm (as are the majority of devices), it will then be prone to the inaccuracy induced by miscuffing, whereby a cuff containing a bladder that is either too long or too short relative to arm circumference is used.

A review of the literature on the century-old controversy relating to the error that may be introduced to blood pressure measurement by using a cuff with a bladder of inappropriate dimensions for the arm for which it is intended has shown that miscuffing is a serious source of error, which must inevitably lead to incorrect diagnosis in practice and erroneous conclusions in hypertension research.[4] There is unequivocal evidence that either too narrow or too short a bladder (undercuffing) will cause overestimation of blood pressure, so-called "cuff hypertension", and there is growing evidence that too wide or too long a bladder (overcuffing) may cause underestimation of blood pressure. Undercuffing has the effect in clinical practice of overdiagnosing hypertension and overcuffing leads to hypertensive subjects being diagnosed as normotensive. Either eventuality has serious implications for the epidemiology of hypertension and clinical practice.

A review of the literature shows that a number of approaches have been used over the years to cope with the difficulty of mismatching and none has been ideal. These have included application of correction factors, a range of cuffs, cuffs containing a variety of bladders, and a cuff for the majority of arms.

Blood pressure measurement in special subjects

Certain groups of people merit special consideration for blood pressure measurement, either because of age, body habitus, or disturbances of blood pressure related to haemodynamic alterations in other parts of the cardiovascular system. Although there is evidence that many subgroups of the hypertensive population may have peculiarities affecting the accuracy of measurement, such as patients with renal disease, patients with diabetes mellitus, women with pre-eclampsia and youths with "spurious" hypertension, discussion will be confined to children, the elderly, obese subjects, and pregnant women.

Children

Blood pressure measurement in children presents a number of difficulties and variability of blood pressure is greater than in adults, and thus any one reading is less likely to represent the true blood pressure. Also increased variability confers a greater tendency for regression towards the mean. Conventional sphygmomanometry is recommended for general use, but systolic pressure is preferred to diastolic pressure because of greater accuracy and reproducibility. Cuff dimensions are most important and three cuffs with bladders measuring 4 × 13 cm, 10 × 18 cm, and the adult dimensions 12 × 26 cm are required for the range of arm sizes likely to be encountered in the age range 0–14 years. The widest cuff practicable should be used. Korotkoff sounds are not reliably audible in all children under one year and in many under five years of age.

Mismatching of bladder and arm
• Bladder too small   Overestimation of BP *Undercuffing*
• Bladder too large   Underestimation of BP *Overcuffing*
Undercuffing more common than *Overcuffing*

Table 5.1 Recommended bladder dimensions. Data reproduced from O'Brien E, Petrie J, Littler WA *et al.* Blood Pressure Measurement: Recommendations of the British Hypertension Society. London: BMJ Books, 1997.

Dimensions (cm)	Subject	Maximum arm circumference (cm)
4 × 13	Small children	17
10 × 18	Medium sized children	
	Lean adults	26
12 × 26	Majority of adult arms	33
12 × 40	Obese adults	50

Accurate readings may be obtained in adults with arm circumferences greater than 50 cm by placing a cuff with a 40 cm bladder so that the centre of the bladder is over the brachial artery. All dimensions have a tolerance of ±1 cm.

A proposal for the future – the "Adjustable Cuff"
On the basis of a thorough examination of the literature and aware of the advances in cuff design, the design features for an "Adjustable Cuff", which would be applicable to all adult arms, have been proposed,[4] and one such cuff is presently undergoing testing (AC Cosor and Sons Ltd (Surgical), London, UK).

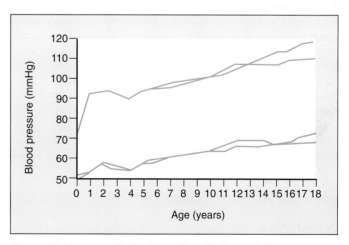

Figure 5.9 Mean systolic (top) and diastolic (bottom) blood pressures of boys and girls from birth to 18 years. Diastolic blood pressure reflects the use of phase IV Korotkov sounds. Reproduced with permission from de Swiet M, Dillon MJ, Littler W, O'Brien E, Padfield PL, Petrie JC. Measurement of blood pressure in children. Recommendations of a working party of the British Hypertension Society. *BMJ* 1989;**299**:469–70.

In such cases conventional sphygmomanometry is impossible and more sensitive methods of detection such as Doppler, ultrasound or oscillometry must be used.[5]

Elderly people

In epidemiological and interventional studies blood pressure predicts morbidity and mortality in elderly people as effectively as in the young.[6] The extent to which blood pressure predicts outcome may be influenced by various factors that affect the accuracy of blood pressure measurement and the extent to which casual blood pressure represents the blood pressure load on the heart and circulation.[7]

The elderly are subject to considerable blood pressure variability, which can lead to a number of circadian blood pressure patterns that are best identified using ambulatory blood pressure measurement. The practical clinical consequence of these variable patterns in the elderly is that blood pressure measuring techniques can be inaccurate and/or misleading.

Pseudohypertension

It has been postulated that as a consequence of the decrease in arterial compliance and arterial stiffening with ageing, indirect sphygmomanometry becomes inaccurate. This has led to the concept of "pseudohypertension" to describe patients with a large discrepancy between cuff and direct blood pressure measurement.[8] The significance of this phenomenon has been disputed,[9] but in elderly patients in whom blood pressure measured with the conventional technique seems to be out of proportion to the clinical findings, referral to a specialist cardiovascular centre for further investigation may be appropriate.

Overweight people

The association between obesity and hypertension has been known since 1923. The link has been confirmed in many epidemiological studies, and has at least two components.[10] Firstly, there appears to be a pathophysiological connection and it may well be that in some cases the two conditions are causally linked, and secondly, if not taken into account, it may result in inaccurate blood pressure values being obtained by indirect measurement techniques.

Obesity may affect the accuracy of blood pressure measurement in children, young people, the elderly, and pregnant women.

The relationship of arm circumference and bladder dimensions has been discussed above. If the bladder is too short, blood pressure will be overestimated—"cuff hypertension"—and, if too long, blood pressure may be underestimated.[4]

Arrhythmias

The difficulty in measuring blood pressure in patients with arrhythmias is that when cardiac rhythm is irregular there is a large variation in blood pressure from beat to beat. Thus in arrhythmias, such as atrial fibrillation, stroke volume and as a consequence blood pressure vary, depending on the preceding pulse interval. Secondly, in such circumstances, there is no

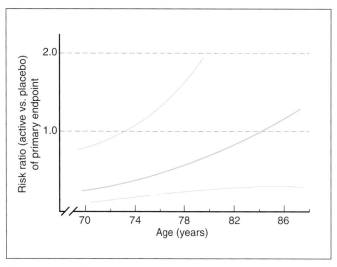

Figure 5.10 Epidemiological graph for the risk of hypertension in the elderly. Reproduced with permission from Dahloff B, Lindholm LH, Hansson L, Schersten B, Ekbom T, Wester PO. Morbidity and mortality in the Swedish Trial in Old Patients with Hypertension (STOP-Hypertension). *Lancet* 1991;**394**:405–12.

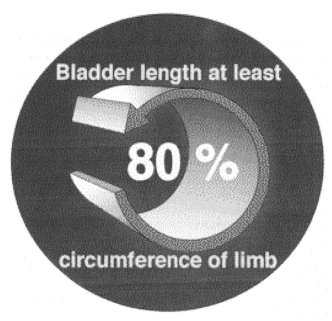

Figure 5.11 Recommended bladder length

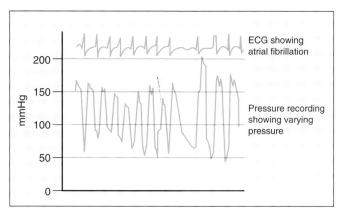

Figure 5.12 Blood pressure in atrial fibrillation

generally accepted method of determining auscultatory endpoints. Furthermore blood pressure measuring devices vary greatly in their ability to accurately record blood pressure in patients with atrial fibrillation, indicating that devices should be validated independently in patients with arrhythmias.[11]

In bradyarrhythmias there may be two sources of error. Firstly, if the rhythm is irregular the same problems as with atrial fibrillation will apply. Secondly, when the heart rate is extremely slow, for example 40 beats per minute, it is important that the deflation rate used is less than for normal heart rates as too rapid deflation will lead to underestimation of systolic and overestimation of diastolic pressure.

Pregnancy

Clinically relevant hypertension occurs in more than 10% of pregnant women in most populations, and in a significant number of these raised blood pressure is a key factor in medical decision making in the pregnancy. Particular attention must be paid to blood pressure measurement in pregnancy because of the important implications for patient management, as well as the fact that it presents some special problems (see also Chapter 12).[12]

There has been much controversy as to whether the muffling or disappearance of sounds should be taken for diastolic blood pressure. The general consensus from obstetricians based on careful analysis of the evidence is that disappearance of sounds (fifth phase) is the most accurate measurement of diastolic pressure, with the proviso that in those rare instances in which sounds persist to zero the fourth phase of muffling of sounds should be used.[13,14]

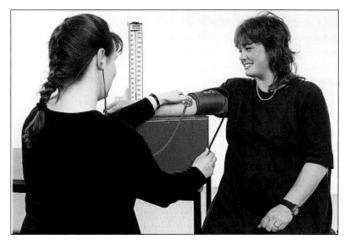

Figure 5.13 Taking blood pressure of a pregnant woman.

References

1 O'Brien E, Owens P. Classic sphygmomanometry: a *fin de siecle* reappraisal. In: *Epidemiology of hypertension*. Bulpitt C, ed. *Handbook of hypertension*. Elsevier: Amsterdam, 2000:130–51.

2 O'Brien E, Petrie J, Littler WA, de Swiet M, Padfield PD, Dillon MJ, Coats A, Mee F. *Blood pressure measurement: recommendations of the British Hypertension Society*. London: BMJ Publishing Group, Third edition, 1997.

3 The British Hypertension Society. *Blood pressure measurement CD ROM*. London: BMJ Books, 1998.

4 O'Brien E. A century of confusion: which bladder for accurate blood pressure measurement? *J Hum Hypertension* 1996;**10**:565–72.

5 de Swiet M, Dillon MJ, Little W, O'Brien E, Padfield PL, Petrie JC. Measurement of blood pressure in children. Recommendations of a working party of the British Hypertension Society. *BMJ* 1989;**299**:497.

6 Dahloff B, Lindholm LH, Hansson L, Schersten B, Ekbom T, Wester PO. Morbidity and mortality in the Swedish Trial in Old Patients with Hypertension (STOP-Hypertension). *Lancet* 1991;**394**:405–12.

7 O'Brien E, O'Malley K. Blood pressure measurement in the elderly with special reference to ambulatory blood pressure measurement. In: *Hypertension in the elderly*. Leonetti G, Cuspedi C, ed. Dordrecht: Kluwer, 1994:13–25.

8 Spence JD, Sibbald WJ, Cape RD. Pseudohypertension in the elderly. *Clin Sci Mol Biol* 1978;**55**:399s–402s.

9 O'Callaghan WG, Fitzgerald D, O'Malley K, O'Brien E. Accuracy of indirect blood pressure measurement in the elderly. *BMJ* 1983;**286**:1545–6.

10 Staessen J, Fagard R, Amery A. The relationship between body weight and blood pressure. *J Hum Hypertens* 1988;**2**:207–17.

11 Stewart MJ, Gough K, Padfield PL. The accuracy of automated blood pressure measuring devices in patients with controlled atrial fibrillation. *J Hypertens* 1995;**13**:297–300.

12 Shennan AH, Halligan AWF. Measuring blood pressure in normal and hypertensive pregnancy. *Baillière's Clinical Obstetrics and Gynaecology* 1999;**13**:1–26.

13 Shennan A, Gupta M, Halligan A, Taylor DJ, de Swiet M. Lack of reproducibility in pregnancy of Korotkoff phase IV as measured by sphygmomanometry. *Lancet* 1996;**347**:139–42.

14 de Swiet M. K5 rather then K4 for diastolic blood pressure measurement in pregnancy. *Hypertension in Pregnancy* 1999;**18**:iii–v.

Part II Conventional sphygmomanometry: technique of auscultatory blood pressure measurement

The measurement of blood pressure in clinical practice by the century-old technique of Riva-Rocci/Korotkoff is dependent on the accurate transmission and interpretation of a signal (Korotkoff sound or pulse wave) from a subject via a device (the sphygmomanometer) to an observer. Errors in measurement can occur at each of these interactionary points of the technique, but by far the most fallible component is the observer.

Observer error

In 1964, Geoffrey Rose and his colleagues classified observer error into three categories.[1]

Systematic error

This leads to both intraobserver and interobserver error. It may be caused by lack of concentration, poor hearing, confusion of auditory and visual cues, etc. The most important factor is failure to interpret the Korotkoff sounds accurately, especially for diastolic pressure.

Rose classification of observer error

- Systematic error
- Terminal digit preference
- Observer prejudice

Observer training techniques

- Direct instruction by an experienced observer
- Instruction manuals and booklets
- Audiotapes
- Video films
- CD-ROM presentations

Recommendations on blood pressure measurement

- 1904: Janeway TC. *The clinical study of blood-pressure*. New York and London: D Appleton.
- 1918: Faught FA. *Blood-pressure primer: the sphygmomanometer and its practical application*. Philadelphia: GP Pilling.
- 1926: Halls Dally JF. *High blood pressure: its variations and control*. London: W Heinemann.
- 1939: *Joint recommendations of the American Heart Association and the Cardiac Society of Great Britain and Ireland: standardization of blood pressure readings*. American Heart Association.
- 1968: Pickering G. *High blood pressure*. London: J & A Churchill.
- 1970: Geddes LA. *The direct and indirect measurement of blood pressure*. Chicago: Year Book Medical Publishers.
- 1981: O'Brien E, O'Malley K, eds. Blood pressure measurement: technique. In: *ABC of Hypertension*. London: BMJ Publishing Group.
- 1981: O'Brien E, O'Malley K. *Essentials of blood pressure measurement*. Edinburgh: Churchill Livingstone.
- 1984: German Hypertension League. *Recommendations for blood pressure measurement [in German]*. Heidelberg: German Hypertension League.
- 1986: Petrie JC, O'Brien ET, Littler WA, de Swiet M. Recommendations on blood pressure measurement. British Hypertension Society. *BMJ* 1986;**293**:611–15.
- 1988: Frohlich ED, Grim C, Labarthe DR, Maxwell MH, Perloff D, Weidman WH. Report of a Special Task Force Appointed by the Steering Committee, American Heart Association. Recommendations for the human blood pressure determination by sphygmomanometers. *Hypertension* 1988;**11**:209A–22A.
- 1988: The Joint National Committee on the Detection, Evaluation, and Treatment of High Blood Pressure. The 1988 report of the Joint National Committee on the Detection, Evaluation, and Treatment of High Blood Pressure. *Arch Intern Med* 1988;**148**:1023–38.
- 1995: Pickering T for an American Society of Hypertension Ad Hoc panel. Recommendations for the use of home(self) and ambulatory blood pressure monitoring. *Am J Hypertens* 1995;**9**:1–11.
- 1997: The Joint National Committee of Prevention, Detection, Evaluation, and Treatment of High Blood Pressure. The sixth report of the Joint National Committee on Prevention, Detection, Evaluation and Treatment of High Blood Pressure. *Arch Intern Med* 1997;**157**:2433–46.
- 1997: O'Brien E, Petrie J, Littler WA, de Swiet M, Padfield PD, Dillon MJ, Coats A, Mee F. *Blood Pressure Measurement: Recommendations of the British Hypertension Society*. BMJ Publishing Group, Third edition, 1997.
- 1999: Guidelines Subcommittee of the World Health Organisation – International Society of Hypertension (WHO-ISH). 1999 World Health Organisation-International Society of Hypertension Guidelines for the management of hypertension. *J Hypertens* 1999;**17**:151–83.
- 1999: Ramsay LE, Williams B, Johnston GD, MacGregor GA, Poston L, Potter JF, Poulter NR, Russell G. Guidelines for management of hypertension: report of the third working party of the British Hypertension Society. *J Hum Hypertens* 1999;**13**:569–92.
- 2000: O'Brien E, Coats A, Owens P, Petrie J, Padheld P, Littler WA, de Swiet MA, Mee F. Use and interpretation of ambulatory blood pressure monitoring: recommendations of the British Hypertension Society. *BMJ* 2000;**320**:1128–34.
- 2000: Asmar R, Zanchetti A on behalf of the Organizing Committee and participants. Guidelines for the use of self-blood pressure monitoring: a summary report of the first international consensus international conference. *J Hypertens* 2000;**18**:493–508.

Terminal digit preference

This refers to the phenomenon whereby the observer rounds off the pressure reading to a digit of his or her choosing, most often to zero. Doctors may have a 12-fold bias in favour of the terminal digit zero; this has grave implications for decisions on diagnosis and treatment, although its greatest effect is in epidemiological and research studies in which it can distort the frequency distribution curve and reduce the power of statistical tests.[2]

Observer prejudice or bias

This is the practice whereby the observer simply adjusts the pressure to meet his or her preconceived notion of what the pressure should be. It usually occurs when there has been recording of an excess of pressures below the cut-off point for hypertension and it reflects the observer's reluctance to diagnose hypertension. This is most likely to occur when an arbitrary division is applied between normal and high blood pressure, for example 140/90 mmHg. An observer might tend to record a favourable measurement in a young healthy man with a borderline increase in pressure, but categorise as hypertensive an obese, middle aged man with a similar reading. Likewise, there might be observer bias in overreading blood pressure to facilitate recruitment for a research project, such as a drug trial. Observer prejudice is a serious source of inaccuracy, as the error cannot usually be demonstrated.[3]

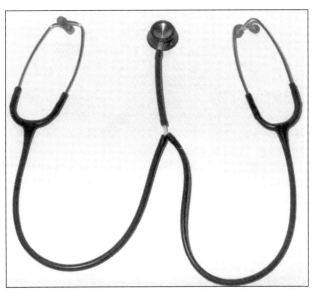

Figure 5.14 Binaural stethoscope

Overcoming error by observer training

The technique of auscultatory blood pressure measurement is a complicated one that is often taken for granted. Instruction to medical students and nurses has not always been as comprehensive as it might be, and assessment for competence in measuring blood pressure has been a relatively recent development.[4] Ironically, these methods of achieving much needed improvement in performing the auscultatory technique have arrived as the mercury sphygmomanometer is under threat and as automated devices move in to replace the observer; these have included: direct instruction using a binaural stethoscope; the use of manuals, booklets and published recommendations; audiotape training methods; videofilm methods, and, most recently, CD-ROM methods. The CD-ROM produced by the Working Party on Blood Pressure Measurement of the British Hypertension Society in 1998[5] incorporates instruction, with examples of blood pressure measurement using a falling mercury column with Korotkoff sounds and a means for the student to assess competence in the technique using a series of examples. The CD is accompanied by the British Hypertension Society booklet *Blood pressure measurement: recommendations of the British Hypertension Society*.[6]

Overcoming error with instrumentation

As mentioned earlier, blood pressure measurement is subject to observer prejudice and terminal digit preference, introducing an error that is unacceptable for research work. Careful training of observers can reduce but not abolish these sources of error, some of which cannot be easily demonstrated. Because accuracy of measurement is particularly desirable in research, efforts have been made to devise devices that would minimise or abolish observer error.

Recommendations for observer training

Training observers in clinical practice: nursing and medical students, doctors, paramedical personnel
- Instruction in the theory of hypertension and blood pressure measurement
- Booklet for reading, e.g. BHS *Recommendations on blood pressure measurement*
- Tutorial sessions with demonstrations using a binaural or multiaural stethoscope
- CD-ROM demonstration using, e.g., the BHS CD-ROM
- CD-ROM assessment
- Repeat CD-ROM assessment until level of accuracy achieved
- Reassessment using BHS CD-ROM every two years

Training observers in research
- Measurement of blood pressure—highest possible standard
- Level of accuracy —90% of SBP and DBP within 5 mmHg
  —100% within 10 mmHg of an expert observer
- Instruction in the theory of hypertension and blood pressure measurement
- Audiogram to check auditory acuity
- Booklet for reading, e.g., BHS *Recommendations on blood pressure measurement*
- Tutorial sessions with demonstrations using a binaural or multiaural stethoscope
- CD-ROM demonstration using, e.g., the BHS CD-ROM
- CD-ROM assessment
- Repeat CD-ROM assessment until level of accuracy achieved
- Training and assessment repeated at least every three months

Measuring blood pressure

Assuming the observer has been trained and shown to be proficient in the technique there are then a number of factors that may affect the performance of the technique.[5,6] Some of these factors are described below.

Attitude of observer

Before taking the blood pressure, the observer should be in a comfortable and relaxed position, because if hurried the pressure will be released too rapidly, resulting in underestimation of systolic and overestimation of diastolic pressures. If any interruption occurs the exact measurement may be forgotten and an approximation made, so the blood pressure should always be written down as soon as it has been measured.

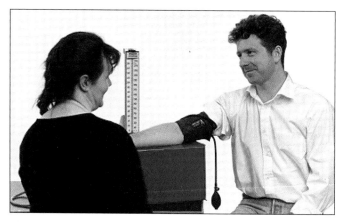

Figure 5.15 Relaxed subject

Mercury and aneroid sphygmomanometers

The mercury sphygmomanometer is a reliable device, but all too often its continuing efficiency has been taken for granted, whereas the aneroid manometer, which is not generally as accurate, is often assumed to be as reliable. These devices have certain features in common; each has an inflation-deflation system, and occluding bladder encased in a cuff, and both devices measure blood pressure by auscultation using a stethoscope.[6]

Inflation-deflation system

The inflation-deflation system consists of an inflating and deflating mechanism connected by rubber tubing to an occluding bladder. The standard mercury and aneroid sphygmomanometers used in clinical practice are operated manually, with inflation being effected by means of a bulb compressed by hand and deflation by means of a release valve, which is also controlled by hand. The pump and control valve are connected to the inflatable bladder and thence to the sphygmomanometer by rubber tubing.

Figure 5.16 Mercury sphygmomanometer

Rubber tubing

Leaks due to cracked or perished rubber make accurate measurement of blood pressure difficult because the fall in mercury cannot be controlled. The rubber should be in a good condition and free from leaks. The minimum length of tubing between the cuff and the manometer should be 70 cm and between the inflation source and the cuff the tubing should be at least 30 cm in length. Connections should be airtight and easily disconnected.

Control valve

One of the most common sources of error in sphygmomanometers is the control valve, especially when an air filter rather than a rubber valve is used. Defective valves cause leakage, making control of pressure release difficult; this leads to underestimation of systolic and overestimation of diastolic pressures. Faults in the control valve may be corrected easily and cheaply, by simply cleaning the filter or replacing the control valve. It is helpful to have a checklist of possible faults and the means of rectifying these.

Consequences of defects in the control valve	
Pumping control valve	little or no effort required
Excessive squeeze on the pump	*filter blocked*
With valve closed	mercury at level steady
Falling mercury	*leak in inflation system*
With valve released	controlled fall of mercury
Failure to control mercury fall	*leak in inflation system*

Hazards of mercury

The mercury sphygmomanometer is a simple and accurate device, which can be easily serviced, but there are rightly concerns about the toxicity of mercury for individuals using mercury sphygmomanometers, and for those who have to service them. Users should be alert therefore to the hazards associated with handling mercury.[7]

However, the greatest concern about mercury is its toxic effects on the environment. Why, we might ask, should we not continue using the mercury sphygmomanometer, which has served us well for the past hundred years? The call to have mercury removed from hospitals comes from the environmental lobby, which, quite correctly, sees mercury as a toxic, persistent and bioaccumable substance. What happens, they ask, to the many tons of mercury supplied for the manufacture of sphygmomanometers and then distributed throughout the world to hospitals and countless individual doctors? Quite simply it finds its way back into the environment through evaporation, sewage or in solid waste, most seriously damaging the marine environment, and it accumulates in soil and in sediments thereby entering the food chain.

The mercury thermometer has been replaced in many countries, and in Sweden and the Netherlands the use of mercury is no longer permitted in hospitals. However, in other European countries, including the UK and Ireland, the move to ban mercury from hospital use has not been received with enthusiasm on the grounds that there is no accurate alternative device to the mercury sphygmomanometer. None the less, the fear of mercury toxicity is making it difficult to get mercury sphygmomanometers serviced, and the precautions recommended for dealing with a mercury spill are influencing purchasing decisions. Indeed, this is what central governmental policy in many countries would favour – the gradual disappearance of mercury from hospitals should a ban become operative.[8-10]

Replacement of the millimetre of mercury with the kilopascal

Banning mercury from the wards raises another issue, which may be of even greater importance for clinical medicine. If the millimetre of mercury is no longer the unit of measurement for blood pressure, there can be no scientific argument against its replacement with the Système International (SI) unit, the kilopascal, which is the accepted unit of pressure measurement in science.[11] If we look back 20 years or so when it was mooted that the kilopascal should become the measure of pressure in medicine, there was an indignant outcry from doctors who claimed that the confusion resulting from such a change of unitage would be unacceptable. They won the day, but on the understanding that the moratorium would last only until such time as a suitable replacement could be found for the mercury sphygmomanometer. So it would seem that when the mercury sphygmomanometer goes, the mainstay of the medical argument for retaining the millimetre of mercury as a unit of measurement, namely that we measure what we see, will also disappear.

Advice to be included in the instructions accompanying a sphygmomanometer using a mercury manometer (from European Standard EN 1060-2)

B.1 Guidelines and precautions
A mercury-type sphygmomanometer should be handled with care. In particular, care should be taken to avoid dropping the instrument or treating it in any way that could result in damage to the manometer. Regular checks should be made to ensure that there are no leaks from the inflation system and to ensure that the manometer has not been damaged so as to cause a loss of mercury.

B.2 Health and safety when handling mercury
Exposure to mercury can have serious toxicological effects; absorption of mercury results in neuropsychiatric disorders and, in extreme cases, of nephrosis. Therefore precautions should be taken when carrying out any maintenance to a mercury-type sphygmomanometer.

When cleaning or repairing the instrument, it should be placed on a tray having a smooth, impervious surface which slopes away from the operator at about 10° to the horizontal, with a water-filled trough at the rear. Suitable gloves (e.g. of latex) should be worn to avoid direct skin contact. Work should be carried out in a well-ventilated area, and ingestion and inhalation of the vapour should be avoided.

For more extensive repairs, the instrument should be securely packed with adequate packing, sealed in a plastic bag or container, and returned to a specialist repairer. It is essential that a high standard of occupational hygiene is maintained in premises where mercury-containing instruments are repaired. Chronic mercury absorption is known to have occurred in individuals repairing sphygmomanometers.

B.3 Mercury spillage
When dealing with a mercury spillage, wear latex gloves. Avoid prolonged inhalation of mercury vapour. Do not use an open vacuum system to aid collection. Collect all the small droplets of spilt mercury into one globule and immediately transfer all the mercury into a container, which should then be sealed.

After removal of as much of the mercury as practicable, treat the contaminated surfaces with a wash composed of equal parts of calcium hydroxide and powdered sulfur mixed with water to form a thin paste. Apply this paste to all the contaminated surfaces and allow to dry. After 24 h, remove the paste and wash the surfaces with clean water. Allow to dry and ventilate the area.

B.4 Cleaning the manometer tube
To obtain the best results from a mercury-type sphygmomanometer, the manometer tube should be cleaned at regular intervals (e.g. under the recommended maintenance schedule). This will ensure that the mercury can move up and down the tube freely, and respond quickly to changes in pressure in the cuff.

During cleaning, care should be taken to avoid the contamination of clothing. Any material contaminated with mercury should be sealed in a plastic bag before disposal in a refuse receptacle.

Preparing for the demise of the mercury sphygmomanometer

Although it will be some years before any move is made to replace the millimetre of mercury, we must prepare for changes in clinical sphygmomanometry. Several simple measures can be instigated immediately. Health care providers are being encouraged to phase out mercury sphygmomanometers and replace them only with devices that have been independently validated against the relevant protocols. Automated devices should provide blood pressures in both millimetres of mercury and kilopascals, so that users can become familiar with kilopascals. Finally, the medical and nursing professions, which constitute the clinical market for blood pressure measuring devices, must ensure that manufacturers provide us with accurate devices designed to our specifications, rather than accepting, as we have done in the past, devices in which these considerations are secondary to the commercial success of the product.[12]

Aneroid manometers

Aneroid sphygmomanometers register pressure through a bellows and lever system, which is mechanically more intricate than the mercury reservoir and column. The jolts and bumps of everyday use affect their accuracy; they lose accuracy over time usually leading to falsely low readings with the consequent underestimation of blood pressure. They are therefore less accurate in use than mercury sphygmomanometers. When calibrated against a mercury sphygmomanometer a mean difference of 3 mmHg is considered to be acceptable; however, 58% of aneroid sphygmomanometers have been shown to have errors greater than 4 mmHg, with about one third of these having errors higher than 7 mmHg.[13] Moreover, aneroid sphygmomanometry is prone to all the problems of the auscultatory technique, namely observer bias and terminal digit preference.

Table of equivalence of units	
mmHg	*kPa*
1	0.1
2	0.2
3	0.4
4	0.6
5	0.7
6	0.8
7	0.9
8	1.0
9	1.2
10	1.4
20	2.6
30	4.0
40	5.4
50	6.7
60	8.0
70	9.4
80	10.7
90	12.0
100	13.4
110	14.7
120	16.0
130	17.4
140	18.7
150	20.0
160	21.4
170	22.7
180	24.0
190	25.4
200	26.7
250	33.4
260	34.7
270	36.0
280	37.4
290	38.7
300	40.0

Shaded areas = decision pressures; kPa rounded to nearest decimal point; 1 mmHg = 0.133 kPa exactly; 1 kPa ~ 8 mmHg; Current scale markings of 2 mmHg ~ 0.25 kPa

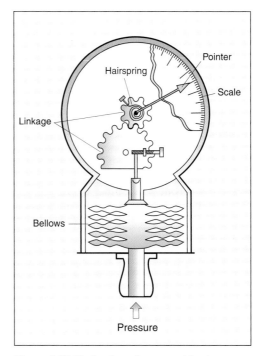

Figure 5.17 Mechanism of an aneroid sphygmomanometer

Position of manometer

The observer should take care when positioning the manometer:
- The manometer should be no further than three feet (92 cm) away so that the scale can be read easily.
- The mercury column should be vertical (some models are designed with a tilt) and at eye level – this is achieved most effectively with stand mounted models, which can be easily adjusted to suit the height of the observer.
- The mercury manometer has a vertical scale and errors will occur unless the eye is kept close to the level of the meniscus. The aneroid scale is a composite of vertical and horizontal divisions and numbers, and must be viewed straight on with the eye on a line perpendicular to the centre of the face of the gauge.

Placing the cuff

The cuff should be wrapped around the arm ensuring that the bladder dimensions are accurate. If the bladder does not completely encircle the arm its centre must be over the brachial artery. The rubber tubes from the bladder are usually placed inferiorly, often at the site of the brachial artery, but it is now recommended that they should be placed superiorly or, with completely encircling bladders, posteriorly, so that the antecubital fossa is easily accessible for auscultation. The lower edge of the cuff should be 2–3 cm above the point of brachial artery pulsation.

Palpatory estimation of blood pressure

The brachial artery should be palpated while the cuff is rapidly inflated to about 30 mmHg above the point where the pulse disappears; the cuff is then slowly deflated, and the observer notes the pressure at which the pulse reappears. This is the approximate level of the systolic pressure. Palpatory estimation is important because Phase I sounds sometimes disappear as pressure is reduced and reappear at a lower level (the auscultatory gap), resulting in systolic pressure being underestimated unless already determined by palpation. The palpatory technique is useful in patients in whom auscultatory endpoints may be difficult to judge accurately – for example, pregnant women, patients in shock, or those taking exercise. (The radial artery is often used for palpatory estimation of the systolic pressure, but by using the brachial artery the observer also establishes its location before auscultation.)

Auscultatory measurement of systolic and diastolic pressures

- Place the stethoscope gently over the brachial artery at the point of maximal pulsation; a bell end-piece gives better sound reproduction, but in clinical practice a diaphragm is easier to secure with the fingers of one hand and covers a larger area.
- The stethoscope should be held firmly and evenly but without excessive pressure – too much pressure might distort the artery, producing sounds below diastolic pressure. The stethoscope end-piece should not touch the clothing, cuff, or rubber tubes to avoid friction sounds.
- The cuff should then be inflated rapidly to about

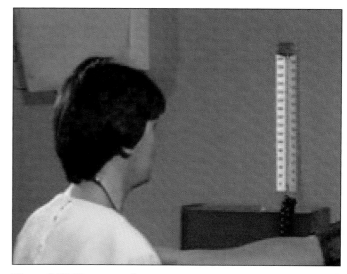

Figure 5.18 Observer and manometer

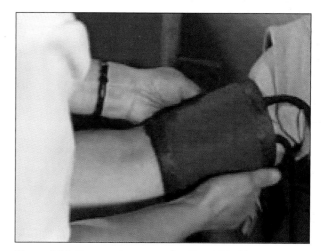

Figure 5.19 Correct placement of cuff and bladder

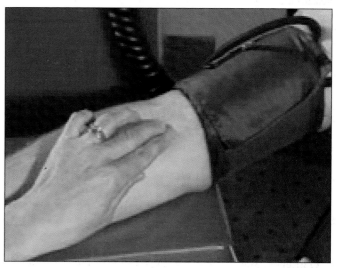

Figure 5.20 Palpating artery

30 mmHg above the palpated systolic pressure and deflated at a rate of 2–3 mmHg per pulse beat (or per second), during which the auscultatory phenomena will be heard.

- When all sounds have disappeared the cuff should be deflated rapidly and completely before repeating the measurement to prevent venous congestion of the arm. The phases shown in the box, which were first described by Nicolai Korotkoff and later elaborated by Witold Ettinger, can be heard.[14]

Diastolic dilemma

For many years recommendations on blood pressure measurement have been uncertain about the diastolic endpoint – the so-called diastolic "dilemma". Phase IV (muffling) may coincide with or be as much as 10 mmHg higher than phase V (disappearance), but usually the difference is less than 5 mmHg; phase V correlates best with intra-arterial pressure. There has been resistance to general acceptance of the silent endpoint until recently, because the silent endpoint can be greatly below the muffling of sounds in some groups of patients-children, pregnant women, anaemic or elderly patients. In some patients sounds may even be audible when cuff pressure is deflated to zero. There is now a general consensus that disappearance of sounds (phase V) should be taken as diastolic pressure except in those subjects mentioned above (as originally recommended by Korotkoff in 1910).[14]

Recording blood pressure

The points to be noted when measuring blood pressure are listed in the adjoining box.

Number of measurements

One measurement should be taken carefully at each visit, with a repeat measurement if there is uncertainty or distraction; do not make a number of hurried measurements.

As a result of the variability of measurements of casual blood pressure, decisions based on single measurements will result in erroneous diagnosis and inappropriate management. Reliability of measurements is improved if repeated measurements are made. The alarm reaction to blood pressure measurement may persist after several visits, so for patients in whom sustained increases of blood pressures are being assessed, a number of measurements should be made on different occasions over a number of weeks or months before diagnostic or management decisions are made.

Auscultatory sounds

- *Phase I*—The first appearance of faint, repetitive, clear tapping sounds which gradually increase in intensity for at least two consecutive beats is the systolic blood pressure
- *Phase II*—A brief period may follow during which the sounds soften and acquire a swishing quality
- *Auscultatory gap*—In some patients sounds may disappear altogether for a short time
- *Phase III*—The return of sharper sounds, which become crisper to regain, or even exceed the intensity of phase I sounds. The clinical significance, if any, to phases II and III has not been established
- *Phase IV*—The distinct abrupt muffling of sounds, which become soft and blowing in quality
- *Phase V*—The point at which all sounds finally disappear completely is the diastolic pressure

---

What to note when measuring blood pressure

- The blood pressure should be written down as soon as it has been recorded
- Measurements of systolic and diastolic pressure should be made to the nearest mmHg
- Pressures should not be rounded off to the nearest 5 or 10 mmHg—digit preference
- The arm in which the pressure is being recorded and the position of the subject should be noted
- Pressures should be recorded in both arms on first attendance
- In obese patients the bladder size should be indicated
- If a "standard cuff" containing a bladder with the dimensions 23 × 12 cm has to be used, it is best to state this together with the measurement so that the presence of "cuff hypertension" can be taken into account in diagnostic and management decisions and arrangements can be made for a more accurate measurement
- In clinical practice the diastolic pressure should be recorded as phase V, except in those patients in whom sounds persist greatly below muffling; this should be clearly indicated
- In hypertension research both phases IV and V should be recorded
- If the patient is anxious, restless or distressed a note of this should be made with the blood pressure
- The presence of an auscultatory gap should always be indicated
- In patients taking blood pressure lowering drugs the optimal time for control of blood pressure will depend on the timing of the drugs; when assessing the effect of antihypertensive drugs the time of drug ingestion should be noted in relation to the time of measurement

References

1 Rose G. Standardisation of observers in blood pressure measurement. *Lancet* 1965;**1**:673–4.
2 Keary L, Atkins N, Molloy E, Mee F, O'Brien E. Terminal digit preference and heaping in blood pressure measurement. *J Hum Hypertens* 1998;**12**:787–88.
3 O'Brien E. Conventional blood pressure measurement. In: *Practical management of hypertension.* Birkenhager W, ed. Dordrecht: Kluwer Academic Publishers, 1996:13–22.
4 O'Brien E, Mee F, Atkins N, O'Malley K, Tam S. Training and assessment of observers for blood pressure measurement in hypertension research. *J Hum Hypertens* 1991;**5**:7–10.
5 The British Hypertension Society. *Blood pressure measurement* CD-ROM. London: BMJ Books, 1998.
6 O'Brien E, Petrie J, Littler WA, de Swiet M, Padfield PD, Dillon MJ, Coats A, Mee F. Blood pressure measurement: Recommendations of the British Hypertension Society. London: BMJ Books, Third edition, 1997.
7 European Standard EN 1060-2 (British Standard BSSEN 1060-2: 1996). Specification for non-invasive

sphygmomanometers. Part 2. Supplementary requirements for mechanical sphygmomanometers. 1995. European Commission for Standardisation, Brussels.

8 O'Brien E. Ave atque vale: the centenary of clinical sphygmomanometry. *Lancet* 1996;**348**:1569–70.

9 O'Brien E. Will mercury manometers soon be obsolete? *J Hum Hypertens* 1995;**9**:933–4.

10 O'Brien E. Replacing the mercury sphygmomanometer. *BMJ* 2000;**320**:815–16.

11 O'Brien E. Will the millimetre of mercury be replaced by the kilopascal. *J Hypertens* 1998;**16**:259–61.

12 O'Brien E, Owens P. Classic sphygmomanometry: a *fin de siecle* reappraisal. In: *Epidemiology of hypertension*. Bulpitt C, ed. *Handbook of hypertension*. Amsterdam: Elsevier, 2000:130–51.

13 Burke MJ, Towers HM, O'Malley K, Fitzgerald D, O'Brien E. Sphygmomanometers in hospitals and family practice: problems and recommendations. *BMJ* 1982;**285**:469–71.

14 O'Brien E, Fitzgerald D. The history of indirect blood pressure measurement. In: *Blood pressure measurement*. O'Brien E, O'Malley K, eds. *Handbook of hypertension*. Amsterdam: Elsevier, 1991:1–54.

Part III Automated sphygmomanometry: ambulatory blood pressure measurement

In recent years, the accuracy of the conventional Riva-Rocci/Korotkoff technique of blood pressure measurement has been questioned and efforts have been made to improve the technique with automated devices. In the same period, recognition of the phenomenon of white coat hypertension, whereby some subjects with apparent elevation of blood pressure have normal, or reduced, blood pressures when measurement is repeated away from the medical environment, has focused attention on methods of measurement, which provide profiles of blood pressure behaviour rather than relying on isolated measurements under circumstances that may in themselves influence the level of blood pressure recorded.

These methodologies have included repeated measurements of blood pressure using the traditional technique, self measurement of blood pressure in the home or workplace, and ambulatory blood pressure measurement (ABPM) using innovative automated devices.[1]

Essential messages

- Consider carefully which monitor to buy
- Consider which type of service is best suited to your needs
- Consider analysis and presentation of data
- Exclusion of white coat hypertension is a major indication
- The technique is valuable in the elderly
- The technique is being increasingly used in pregnancy

Setting up an ambulatory blood pressure measurement service

Which monitor to buy?

A large variety of ambulatory blood pressure measurement devices are now available on the market, and the number will increase as the technique of ambulatory blood pressure measurement becomes more widespread. A number of factors should influence this choice, among which the most important is to ensure that the device has been validated independently according to either the protocol of the British Hypertension Society (BHS),[2] and/or that of the Association for the Advancement of Medical Instrumentation (AAMI).[3]

What type of service?

Doctors in practice may establish their own ambulatory blood pressure measurement service, refer patients to a hospital ambulatory blood pressure measurement service, or refer patients to a blood pressure clinic for full evaluation, which includes ambulatory blood pressure measurement. Often the option of an open access referral service is used, with referral of problem or complicated cases for fuller evaluation in a blood pressure clinic.

Training requirements

The technique of ambulatory blood pressure measurement is specialised, and should be approached with the care reserved for any such procedure. An understanding of the principles of traditional blood pressure measurement, cuff fitting, monitor function and analysis and interpretation of ambulatory blood pressure measurement data as presented in the BHS Working Party CD-ROM on blood pressure measurement is recommended.[4] In practice, a nurse with an interest and experience in hypertension can master the use of ambulatory blood pressure measurement devices after relatively brief training. However, the analysis and interpretation of ambulatory blood pressure measurement profiles requires experience in the technique, which is best acquired by the doctor in charge of an ambulatory blood pressure measurement service.

Using an ambulatory blood pressure measurement monitor

Time needs to be given to fitting the monitor and preparing the patient for the monitoring period if good results are to be obtained.[1] The key to successful ambulatory blood pressure measurement is educating the patient in the process of monitoring and instructions should be explained and printed on a diary card. In clinical practice measurements are usually made at half-hourly intervals so as not to interfere with activity during the day and with sleep at night, but measurements can be made more frequently if indicated. There are a number of ways of analysing blood pressures recorded during the 24-hour cycle.[5] One simple and popular method is to assess the time of awakening and sleeping from diary card entries. Another is to use a fixed time method in which the retiring (2101 to 0059 hours) and rising (0601 to 0859 hours) periods during which blood pressures are subject to considerable variation are eliminated, with the daytime period being from 0900 to 2100

Which monitor to choose

- Check for independent validation by BHS/AAMI protocols
- How much will it cost?
- How expensive is the software?
- Is the software what you need?
- Are the instructions adequate?
- How much will maintenance cost?
- How expensive are consumables—batteries, etc.?
- Have you adequate computer facilities?
- Is the technical/nursing back-up available?
- Are training facilities available?
- Is the warranty adequate?
- Is there an adequate servicing facility?

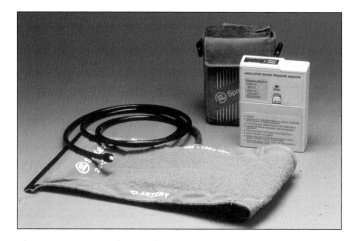

Figure 5.21 SpaceLabs 90207 ABPM monitor

Details of ABPM device manufacturers

Additional information about manufacturers can be found on the *BMJ*'s website: www.bmj.com

---

Using an ambulatory blood pressure monitor

- 15–30 minutes needed
- Relax patient in a quiet room
- Enter patient details into monitor
- Measure BP in both arms
  If SBP difference < 10 mmHg use non-dominant arm
  If SBP difference ≥ 10 mmHg use higher pressure arm
- Select appropriate cuff—see "BHS recommendations on cuff dimensions" below
- Select frequency of measurement—usually every 30 minutes day and night
- Inactivate LCD display
- Give patient written instructions and a diary card
- Instruct patient how to remove and inactivate monitor after 24 hours

Table 5.2 Ambulatory blood pressure measuring devices available on the market which have been subjected to validation by BHS* and AAMI protocols†

Device	AAMI protocol	BHS protocol: systolic/diastolic BP	Circumstance of validation
Accutracker II	Passed	A/C	At rest
CH-DRUCK	Passed	A/A	At rest with pressure ranges
Daypress 500	Passed	A/B	At rest
DIASYS 200	Passed	C/C	At rest
DIASYS Integra	Passed	B/A B/B	At rest with pressure ranges
ES-H531	Passed	A/A B/B	At rest with performance characteristics
Meditech ABPM-04	Passed	B/B	At rest with pressure ranges
Nissei DS-240	Passed	B/A	At rest
OSCILL-IT	Passed	C/B	At rest
Profilomat	Passed	B/A	At rest with pressure ranges
	Passed	B/C	In pregnancy
Profilomat II	SBP fail DBP pass	C/B	At rest with pressure ranges
QuietTrak	Passed	A/A B/B	At rest
	Failed	B/B	In pregnancy
Save 33, Model 2	Passed	B/B	At rest
Schiller BR-102	Passed	B/B	At rest with pressure ranges
SpaceLabs 90202	Passed	B/B	At rest
SpaceLabs 90207	Passed	B/B	At rest with pressure ranges
SpaceLabs 90207	Passed	A/C B/B B/C C/C	In pregnancy
	SBP pass/DBP fail	C/D	In children
	Passed	A/C	In the elderly with postural effect
SpaceLabs 90217	Passed	A/A	At rest with pressure ranges
TM-2420 Model 5	Passed	C/C	At rest
TM-2420 Model 6	Passed	B/B	At rest
TM-2420 Model 7	Passed	B/B	At rest
TM-2421	Passed	B/A	At rest
Takeda 2421	N/A	C/C A/B	In children with postural effect
Takeda 2430	Passed	A/A	At rest with performance characteristics

Grades A–D according to BHS protocol denote agreement with mercury standard: A = best agreement, recommended for clinical use, B = good agreement, recommended for clinical use, C and D = poor and worst agreement, not recommended for clinical use
*Criteria for fulfilment of BHS protocol and recommendation for clinical use: devices must achieve at least grade B/B
†Criteria for fulfilment of AAMI standard and recommendation for clinical use: mean difference ≤ 5 mmHg and SD ≤ 8 mmHg

hours and night-time from 0100 to 0600 hours; in this way the variations that may exist between the young and the old and in different cultures are to some extent eliminated from the analysis.

Presenting the data

Many statistical techniques exist for describing different aspects of ambulatory records, and no one method is ideal.[1] The important points are summarised in the box.

The detection of artefactual readings and the handling of outlying values (which may or may not be erroneous) have been the subject of debate, and if there are sufficient measurements editing is not necessary.

Ambulatory blood pressure measurement devices are usually sold with individual software packages, which present data in a variety of ways. It would facilitate practice if the graphic presentation of ambulatory blood pressure measurement data were standardised, much as is the case for ECG recordings. In other words, the presentation of data would be independent of the type of monitor used. Such a standardised approach might provide a graphic display of ambulatory blood pressure measurement data (on screen or printout) with a visual time/pressure graph with blood pressure plotted on the vertical axis and time on the horizontal axis, and levels of normality can also be shown.[6,7] One program (DABL®, Cardiovascular 2000 ECF Medical, Dublin, Republic of Ireland) provides a printed report derived from the ambulatory blood pressure measurement data.[6]

Instructions for patients

(To be explained to patient and reinforced on an instruction/diary card)
- Explain procedure
- Explain frequency of inflation and deflation
- Explain how to deflate manually
- Explain about failed measurements and what the monitor will do
- Instruct to keep arm steady during measurement
- Instruct to keep arm at heart level during measurement
- Instruct to engage in normal activities between measurements
- Instruct to keep monitor attached at night
- Instruct to place monitor under pillow or on bed at night
- Provide a help-line number for problems or anxiety
- Provide diary card for the following:
    level of activity at time of blood pressure measurement
    time of going to bed
    time of rising
    time of taking medication
    record any symptoms

The issue of normality/abnormality in ambulatory blood pressure measurement is controversial and the approaches to defining normality have been the subject of discussion, but the levels shown in the table below are commonly used.[8] The evidence from on-going longitudinal studies gives some support to lower levels of normality for ambulatory blood pressure measurement, and we appreciate that these levels may be regarded as conservative by some.

Table 5.3 Recommended levels of normality for ambulatory blood pressure measurement

	Normal	*Abnormal*
Daytime	≤ 135/85	> 140/90
Night-time	≤ 120/70	> 125/75
24-hour	≤ 130/80	> 135/85

The evidence supporting these demarcation levels is based on firm evidence from a number of studies; the evidence is not yet available to make recommendations for the intermediate pressure ranges between the "normal" and "abnormal" levels, nor for recommendations lower than those given. It must be emphasised that these levels are only a guide to "normality" and that lower levels may taken as "abnormal" in patients whose total risk factor profile is high, and in whom there is concomitant disease, such as diabetes mellitus.[9]

Presenting the data

- Number of measurements
  Day > 14 SBP and DBP measurements
  Night > 7 SBP and DBP measurements
- Causes of poor ABPM
  Poor technique
  Arrhythmias
  Small pulse volume
  Inability of automated devices to measure blood pressure
- Editing data
  Restrict editing to physiologically impossible pressures, e.g. DBP = SBP
- Displaying data
  Plot data see Figure 5.22
  Statistics to include:
    Mean daytime SBP and DBP and heart rate
    Mean night-time SBP and DBP and heart rate
    Mean 24-hour SBP and DBP and heart rate

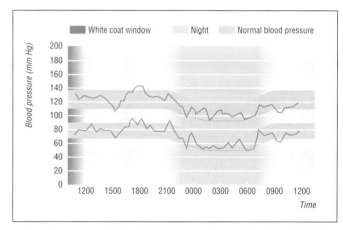

Figure 5.22 Example of a normal ambulatory blood pressure pattern plotted by the DABL® Program.

Clinical indications for ambulatory blood pressure measurement

Ambulatory blood pressure measurement provides a large number of blood pressure measurements over a period of time – usually the 24-hour period – which can be plotted to give a profile of blood pressure behaviour. Although in practice the average day (or night-time) blood pressures are used to govern decisions, the clinical use of ambulatory blood pressure measurement has allowed for a number of phenomena in hypertension to be more clearly identified than is possible with other methods of blood pressure measurement.[7,10] Ambulatory blood pressure measurement can benefit patients with hypertension in the categories in the box.

Possible clinical indications for ambulatory blood pressure measurement

- Exclusion of white coat hypertension
- Deciding diagnosis in borderline hypertension
- Elderly patients for treatment
- To identify nocturnal hypertension
- Hypertensive patients resistant to treatment
- As a guide to antihypertensive drug treatment
- Hypertension of pregnancy
- To diagnose hypotension

Patients with white coat hypertension

From the first use of home and ambulatory monitoring, it became apparent that the clinic or office blood pressure could be elevated over and above the ambulatory mean blood pressure, due to the white coat phenomenon, which may convert ambulant normotensives into clinic hypertensives. The features of white coat hypertension are summarised in the box. In normotensive people daytime ambulatory blood pressure may be a little higher than conventional blood pressure, but in hypertensive subjects daytime blood pressure is usually substantially, but unpredictably, lower than conventional blood pressure.

Patients with clinic borderline hypertension

The same reasoning applies to patients with borderline elevation of blood pressure, especially young subjects, in whom life-long drug therapy may be inappropriately prescribed, and who may be penalised for insurance or employment if the diagnosis of "hypertension" is misapplied.

Elderly patients in whom treatment is being considered

The results of the ambulatory study of the Systolic Hypertension in Europe (SYST-Eur) trial show that systolic blood pressure measured conventionally in the elderly may average 20 mmHg higher than daytime ambulatory blood pressure,[11] thereby leading to inevitable overestimation of isolated systolic hypertension in the elderly and probable excessive treatment of the condition. Moreover, results from this study also show that ambulatory systolic blood pressure was a significant predictor of cardiovascular risk over and above conventional systolic blood pressure. A number of ambulatory patterns are found in the elderly, among which are a number of hypotensive states due to baroreceptor or autonomic failure.[12] As the elderly can be very susceptible to the adverse effects of blood pressure lowering drugs, identification of hypotension becomes particularly important, though its management may present a considerable therapeutic challenge.

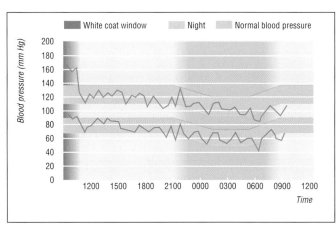

Figure 5.23 White coat hypertension

Features of white coat hypertension

- Definition
  Abnormal office blood pressure ≥ 140/90 mmHg
  Normal daytime ambulatory blood pressure
  < 135/85 mmHg
- Prevalence of white coat hypertension
  15–30% general population
  30% pregnancy
- Risks from white coat hypertension
  Considerably less than sustained hypertension
  Probable small risk compared to normotensives
  Possibly a prehypertensive state?
  Not an entirely innocent condition
- Clinical implications
  No clinical characteristics to assist diagnosis
  Must be considered in newly diagnosed hypertensives
  Should be considered before drug prescribing
  Must be placed in context of overall risk profile
  Reassurance for employment
  Reassurance for insurance and pension liability
  Common in the elderly and pregnancy
  Less drug prescribing
  Need for follow-up and re-monitoring

Ambulatory blood pressure patterns in the elderly

- White coat hypertension
- Isolated systolic hypertension
- Postural hypotension
- Post-prandial hypotension
- Daytime hypotension/nocturnal hypertension
- Drug-induced hypotension
- Autonomic failure

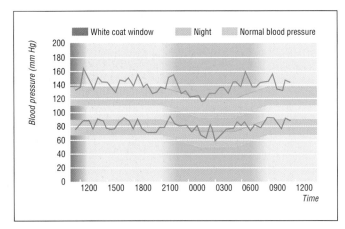

Figure 5.24 Borderline hypertension

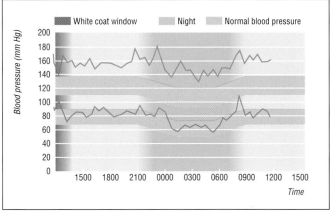

Figure 5.25 Isolated systolic hypertension

Nocturnal hypertension

Ambulatory blood pressure measurement is the only non-invasive blood pressure measuring technique that permits measurement of blood pressure during sleep. The relevance of nocturnal hypertension is still controversial, but there is increasing evidence that night-time blood pressure may provide important information.[13] Nocturnal blood pressure levels, for example, are independently associated with end-organ damage,[14] over and above the risk associated with daytime values. It has also been shown that absence of nocturnal "dipping" of blood pressure to lower levels than during the day is associated with target organ involvement, and may be a useful (though non-specific) clue as to the presence of secondary hypertension.

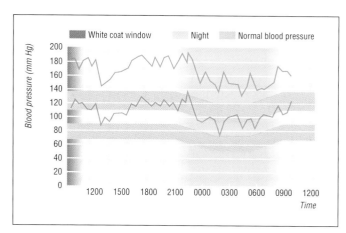

Figure 5.26 Systolic and diastolic hypertension with night-time dip

Patients with resistant hypertension

In patients whose conventional blood pressure remains consistently above 150/90 mmHg in spite of treatment with three antihypertensive drugs, ambulatory blood pressure measurement may indicate that the apparent lack of response is due, in fact, to the white coat phenomenon, or the presence of a non-dipping nocturnal pattern may suggest secondary hypertension.

Ambulatory blood pressure measurement in pregnancy

As in the non-pregnant state, the main use for ambulatory blood pressure measurement in pregnancy is the identification of white coat hypertension, which may occur in nearly 30% of pregnant women.[15] Its recognition is important, so that pregnant women are not admitted to hospital or given antihypertensive drugs unnecessarily or excessively. Normal values for ambulatory blood pressure in the pregnant population are available, and the changes in pressure which occur during the trimesters of pregnancy and in the postpartum period have been defined.[16] The evidence that ambulatory blood pressure measurement may predict pre-eclamptic toxaemia is not yet conclusive. However ambulatory blood pressure correlates better with proteinuria than does conventional sphygmomanometry, it is a better predictor of hypertensive complications, and women diagnosed by the technique as having hypertension have infants with lower birth weight than normotensive women.[16–20] Moreover, women with white coat hypertension tend to have more caesarean sections than normotensive women, suggesting that if ambulatory blood pressure measurement was used to measure blood pressure rather than the conventional technique, caesarean delivery might be avoided.[15]

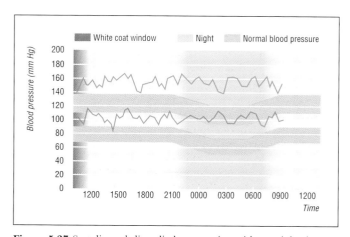

Figure 5.27 Systolic and diastolic hypertension without night-time dip

Ambulatory hypotension

Reference has already been made to the clinical use of ambulatory blood pressure measurement in identifying hypotensive episodes in the elderly, but it may also be used in young patients in whom hypotension is suspected of causing symptoms. Ambulatory blood pressure measurement may also demonstrate drug-induced drops in blood pressure in treated hypertensive patients, which may have untoward effects in patients with a compromised arterial circulation, such as those with coronary and cerebrovascular disease.[21]

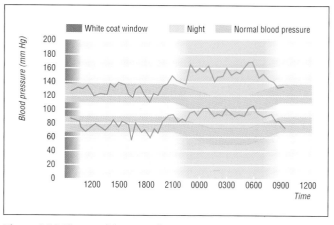

Figure 5.28 Nocturnal hypertension

Ambulatory blood pressure measurement in drug treatment

The role of ambulatory blood pressure measurement in guiding drug treatment is currently the subject of much research, and its role in this regard has not yet been fully established. However, recent reviews of the clinical value of ambulatory blood pressure measurement have highlighted the potential of 24-hour recordings of blood pressure in guiding antihypertensive medication. Furthermore, a recent well controlled study showed that when ambulatory blood pressure measurement was used as the basis for prescribing rather than clinic blood pressure, significantly less antihypertensive medication was prescribed.[22] Quite apart from this attribute, ambulatory blood pressure measurement gives the prescribing doctor an assessment of the response to treatment that conventional measurement cannot provide, the efficacy of treatment without the white coat effect can be ascertained, excessive drug effect and the occurrence of symptoms can be determined, and the duration of drug effect over the 24-hour period can be demonstrated.

Who should be re-monitored?

Ambulatory blood pressure measurement causes inconvenience to patients, and it should be used, therefore, with discretion. The decision as to when to repeat ambulatory blood pressure measurement is largely one of clinical judgment, which may be influenced by factors such as excessive blood pressure variability, an inappropriate response to treatment, an adverse risk factor profile and the need for careful control of blood pressure, such as in hypertensive patients with diabetes mellitus or renal disease. As a general rule it is usually unnecessary to repeat ambulatory blood pressure measurement more frequently than annually.[1] Conventional blood pressure measurement may be relied on for follow-up in patients who do not have a white coat effect on ambulatory blood pressure measurement. The patients in whom re-monitoring may be helpful are listed in the box.

Indications for re-monitoring

Usually annual re-monitoring is sufficient
- Patients with white coat hypertension
- Treated patients with white coat effect
- Elderly patients with hypotension
- Patients with nocturnal hypertension
- Changes in medication

References

1 O'Brien E, Coats A, Owens P, Petrie J, Padheld P, Littler WA, de Swiet MA, Mee F. Use and interpretation of ambulatory blood pressure monitoring: recommendations of the British Hypertension Society. *BMJ* 2000: **320**: 1128–34.

2 O'Brien E, Petrie J, Littler WA *et al.* The British Hypertension Society Protocol for the evaluation of blood pressure measuring devices. *J Hypertens* 1993;**11**(Suppl 2):S43–63.

3 American National Standard for Electronic or Automated Sphygmomanometers: ANSI/AAMI SP10-1987. Arlington, VA: Association for the Advancement of Medical Instrumentation, 1993; p40.

4 The British Hypertension Society. *Blood pressure measurement CD-ROM.* London: BMJ Books, 1998.

5 Fagard R, Staessen J, Thijs L. Optimal definition of daytime and night-time blood pressure. *Blood Press Monitor* 1997;**2**:315–21.

6 Atkins N, O'Brien E. DABL97–a computer program for the assessment of blood pressure, risk factors and cardiovascular target organ involvement in hypertension. *J Hypertens* 1998;**16**(Suppl 2):S198.

7 Owens P, Lyons S, O'Brien E. Ambulatory blood pressure in the hypertensive population; patterns and prevalence of hypertensive sub-forms. *J Hypertens* 1998;**16**:1735–43.

8 O'Brien ET, Staessen J. Normotension and hypertension as defined by 24-hour ambulatory blood pressure monitoring. *Blood Pressure* 1995;**4**:266–82.

9 Ramsay LE, Williams B, Johnston GD, MacGregor GA, Poston L, Potter JF, Poulter NR, Russell G. Guidelines for management of hypertension: report of the third working party of the British Hypertension Society. *J Hum Hypertens* 1999;**13**:569–92.

10 Owens P, Atkins N, O'Brien E. The diagnosis of white coat hypertension by ambulatory blood pressure measurement. *Hypertension* 1999;**34**:267–72.

11 Staessen J, Thijs L, Fagard R, for the Systolic Hypertension in Europe (SYST-Eur) Trial Investigators. Conventional and ambulatory blood pressure as predictors of cardiovascular risk in older patients with systolic hypertension. *J Hypertens* 1999;**17**(Suppl 3):S16.

12 Owens P, O'Brien ET. Hypotension; a forgotten illness? *Blood Press Monitor* 1996;**2**:3–14.

13 O'Brien E, Sheridan J, O'Malley K. Dippers and non-dippers (letter). *Lancet* 1988;**ii**:397.

14 Verdecchia P, Schillaci G, Guerrieri M, Gatteschi C, Benemio G, Boldrini F *et al.* Circadian blood pressure changes and left ventricular hypertrophy in essential hypertension. *Circulation* 1990;**81**:528–36.

15 Bellomo G, Narducci PL, Rondoni F, Pastorelli G, Stagnoni G, Angeli G, Verdecchia P. Prognostic value of 24-hour blood pressure in pregnancy. *JAMA* 1999;**282**:1447–52.

16 Halligan A, O'Brien E, O'Malley K, Mee F, Atkins N, Conroy R, Walshe J, Darling M. Twenty-four hour ambulatory blood pressure measurement in a primigravid population. *J Hypertens* 1993;**11**:869–73.

17 Higgins JR, Walshe JJ, Halligan A, O'Brien E, Conroy R, Darling MR. Can 24 hour ambulatory blood pressure measurement predict the development of hypertension in primigravidae? *Br J Obstet Gynaecol* 1997;**104**:356–62.

18 Halligan AWF, Shennan A, Lambert PC, Taylor DJ, de Swiet M. Automated blood pressure measurement as a predictor of proteinuric pre-eclampsia. *Br J Obstet Gynaecol* 1997;**104**:559–62.

19 Penny JA, Halligan AWF, Shennan AH, Lambert PC, Jones DR, de Swiet M, Taylor DJ. Automated, ambulatory, or conventional blood pressure measurement in pregnancy: which is the better predictor of severe hypertension? *Am J Obstet Gynecol* 1998;**178**:521–6.

20 Churchill D, Perry IJ, Beevers DG. Ambulatory blood pressure in pregnancy and fetal growth. *Lancet* 1997;**349**:7–10.

21 Owens P, O'Brien ET. Hypotension in patients with coronary disease–can profound hypotensive events cause myocardial ischaemic events? *Heart* 1999;**82**:477–81.

22 Staessen JA, Byttebier G, Buntinx F, Celis H, O'Brien E, Fagard R, for the Ambulatory Blood Pressure Monitoring and Treatment Investigators. Antihypertensive treatment based on conventional blood or ambulatory blood pressure measurement. A randomised controlled trial. *JAMA* 1997;**278**:1065–72.

Part IV Automated sphygmomanometry: self blood pressure measurement

It has been recognised for over 50 years that blood pressure measured in the home is lower than that recorded by a doctor.[1] The discrepancy between pressures recorded in the home and the clinic has been confirmed repeatedly, and is present regardless of whether patients, or their relatives or friends, measure blood pressure.[2]

Why then has home measurement of blood pressure failed to achieve the success and popularity of home urinalysis in diabetes? There are a number of explanations: training patients to measure their own blood pressures using the auscultatory technique was troublesome and time consuming and not suitable for many subjects; the technique is subject to bias whereby some patients record pressures of their own making; doctors often perceive the technique as one which induces anxiety or causes the patient to take an obsessional interest in blood pressure; most automated devices available for self measurement had not been validated adequately, or had been shown to be inaccurate; finally, because the technique was little used data has been lacking to provide the evidence needed to assure its place in modern clinical practice.

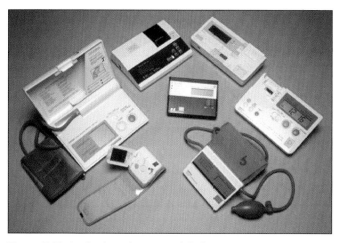

Figure 5.29 A selection of automated devices.

For these reasons home measurement of blood pressure has not received widespread acceptance in medical practice, although its popularity with patients is considerable. However, the advent of accurate inexpensive automated devices which can provide a printout of blood pressure measurement with the time and date of measurement, or which allow storage of data for later analysis, plotting and/or electronic transmission of data, has removed many of the drawbacks referred to above, and there is now a renewed interest in self blood pressure measurement. This revival of interest in an old methodology was recognised when experts from around the world gathered at the First International Consensus Conference on Self-Blood Pressure Measurement (SBPM) in Versailles in 1999 to discuss the evidence for and against the technique and to establish guidelines for its use in clinical medicine.[3-10] One of the recurring themes of the conference was the need for further research to determine the precise role of self measurement in practice.

A number of developments, not least the availability of accurate automated devices, herald the demise of so-called classic sphygmomanometry and the dawning of a new era in blood pressure measurement.

Automated devices: an automated alternative to mercury

Automated devices, by providing timed printouts of blood pressure, remove many of the sources of error associated with the conventional auscultatory technique, and thereby improve the overall accuracy of measurement, provided, of course, that they themselves are accurate. Although the mercury sphygmomanometer is disappearing from use, unfortunately there are not many alternative devices available to replace it. The automated devices on the market have been designed for self measurement of blood pressure, and although automated devices are being developed specifically for clinical use, the automated devices presently being used in clinical practice have been adapted for a use for which they were not designed.

The advent of accurate automated devices, however welcome, is not without problems. Firstly, automated devices have been notorious for their inaccuracy, although accurate devices are now appearing on the market. Secondly, the available automated devices were designed for self-measurement of blood pressure, and it should not be assumed that they will be suitable for clinical use, or that they will remain accurate with use, although some are being used successfully in hospital practice and a number of major hypertension studies. Thirdly, oscillometric techniques cannot measure blood pressure in all situations, particularly in patients with arrhythmias, such as rapid atrial fibrillation, and there are also individuals in whom these devices cannot measure blood pressure for reasons that are not always apparent. Fourthly, doctors are uneasy about trusting algorithmic methods, zealously guarded by manufacturers. To ensure that new devices conform with recommended validation protocols the mercury sphygmomanometer will have to be retained as a gold standard in designated laboratories.[11]

Topics addressed at the First International Consensus Conference on Self Blood Pressure Measurement in 1999

1. Devices and validation
2. Normal values
3. Procedure for the user
4. Usefulness of self BP measurement in the diagnosis of hypertension
5. Prognostic value of self BP measurement
6. Applications of self BP measurement in therapy and clinical trials

Publications relating to validation procedures and the application of validation protocols to assessing the overall accuracy of available blood pressure measuring devices. Publications relating to individual device validation are not listed but nearly all such published validation studies have been performed according to the BHS and/or AAMI protocols.

1987 American National Standard for Electronic or Automated Sphygmomanometers. ANSI/AAMI SP10-1987. Association for the Advancement of Medical Instrumentation. 3330 Washington Boulevard, Suite 400, Arlington, VA 22201-4598. USA.1987. Pp. 25.

1989 Australian Standard: Sphygmomanometers. AS 3655-1989. Standards Australia. Standards Association of Australia. Standards House, 80 Arthur St., N. Sydney, New South Wales. 1989. Pp. 36.

1990 O'Brien E, Petrie J, Littler WA, Padfield PL, O'Malley K, Jamieson M, Altman D, Bland M, Atkins N. British Hypertension Protocol: Evaluation of automated and semi-automated blood pressure measuring devices with special reference to ambulatory systems. *J Hypertens* 1990;**8**:607–619.

1993 O'Brien E, Petrie J, Littler WA *et al.* The British Hypertension Society Protocol for the evaluation of blood pressure measuring devices. *J Hypertens* 1993;**11**(suppl 2):S43–S63. American National Standard. Electronic or automated sphygmomanometers. ANSI/AAMI SP 10-1992. Association for the Advancement of Medical Instrumentation. 3330 Washington Boulevard, Suite 400, Arlington, VA 22201-4598. 1993. Pp. 40.

1994 O'Brien E, Atkins N. A comparison of the BHS and AAMI protocols for validating blood pressure measuring devices: can the two be reconciled? *J Hypertension* 1994;**12**:1089–1094.

1995 O'Brien E, Atkins N, Staessen J. State of the Market: a review of ambulatory blood pressure monitoring devices. *Hypertension* 1995;**26**:835–842. European Standard EN 1060-1 (British Standard BSSEN 1060-1:1996). Specification for Non-invasive sphygmomanometers. Part I. General requirements. 1995. European Commission for Standardisation. Rue Stassart 36, B-1050, Brussels. European Standard EN 1060-2 (British Standard BSSEN 1060-2:1996). Specification for Non-invasive sphygmomanometers. Part 2. Supplementary requirements for mechanical sphygmomanometers. 1995. European Commission for Standardisation. Rue Stassart 36, B-1050 Brussels.

1996 Normenausschuß Feinmechanik und Optik (NaFuO) im DIN Deutsches Institut für Normierung e V: Non-invasive sphygmomanometers – Clinical Investigation. Berlin: Beuth Verlag; 1996.

1997 Non-invasive sphygmomanometers. Part 3. Supplementary requirements for electro-mechanical blood pressure measuring systems. British Standard BS EN 1060-3: 1997. European Standard EN 1060-3 1997. European Committee for Standardization. Central Secretariat: rue de Stassart 36, B-1050, Brussels.

1998 O'Brien E. Automated blood pressure measurement: state of the market in 1998 and the need for an international validation protocol for blood pressure measuring devices. *Blood Pressure Monit* 1998;**3**:205–211.

2000 O'Brien E. Proposals for simplyfing the validation protocols of the British Hypertension Society and the Association for the Advancement of Medical Instrumentation. *Blood Pressure Monit* 2000;**5**:43–45. O'Brien E, Waeber B, Parati G, Staessen G, Myers MG on behalf of the European Society of Hypertension Working Group on Blood Pressure Monitoring. Blood Pressure Measuring Devices: Validated Instruments 2000. *BMJ* In press, 2000.

Table 5.4 Automated blood pressure measuring devices for self measurement of upper arm blood pressure, which have been subjected to validation by the BHS* and AAMI† protocols

Device	AAMI	BHS	Circumstance	Recommendation
Philips HP5332 [26]	Failed	C/A	At rest	Unacceptable for clinical use
Nissei DS-175 [26]	Failed	D/A	At rest	Unacceptable for clinical use
Omron HEM-705CP [26]	Passed	B/A	At rest	Acceptable for clinical use
Omrou HEM 706 [27]	Passed	B/C	At rest	Unacceptable for clinical use
Omron HEM 403C [28]	Failed	C/C	Protocol violation	Unacceptable for clinical use
Omron HEM-703CP [29]	Passed	NA	Intra-arterial	Possibly acceptable for clinical use
Omron M4 [30]	Passed	A/A	Abstract only; detail missing	Possibly acceptable for clinical use
Omron MX2 [30]	Passed	A/A	Abstract only; detail missing	Possibly acceptable for clinical use
Omron HEM-722C [31]	????	A/A	Protocol violation	Possibly acceptable for clinical use
Omron HEM-722C [32]	Passed	A/A	Rest/Elderly	Acceptable for clinical use
Omron HEM-735C [32]	Passed	B/A	Rest/Elderly	Acceptable for clinical use
Ornron HEM-713C [33]	Passed	B/B	At rest	Acceptable for clinical use
Omron HEM-737 Intellisense [34]	Passed	B/B	At rest	Acceptable for clinical use

See notes to Table 5.2.

Device accuracy: validation requirements for sphygmomanometers

Manufacturing blood pressure measuring devices is big business. In Germany, for example, 1.2 million wrist devices for self measurement of blood pressure are sold annually.[11] Only a fraction of the many hundreds of models available worldwide have been subjected to independent validation, but it does not necessarily follow that the consumers who constitute the large market from which manufacturers may profit are well served by their suppliers, and this includes medical as well as non-medical consumers. As the professional consumers we have an obligation to ensure that when blood pressure is measured, the readings obtained are accurate and a true reflection of the haemodynamic state. If this basic principle is ignored our patients will be subject to inaccurate diagnosis and inappropriate management, which may involve inadequate drug treatment, on the one hand, or unnecessary drug treatment for life on the other. Hence, in the last decade or so, much attention has been given to validating blood pressure measuring devices for accuracy independently of the sometimes extravagant claims made by manufacturers for their products. There are two published standards for the evaluation of blood pressure measuring devices – the American Association for the Advancement of Medical Instrumentation (AAMI) Standard,[12] which is accepted by the Food and Drug Administration as the national standard in the United States, and the more comprehensive protocol of the British Hypertension Society (BHS).[13] In brief these protocols compare an ABPM device against the traditional auscultatory technique of blood pressure measurement in normotensive and hypertensive subjects with a wide range of blood pressures, and in varying age groups. On the basis of these results, the protocols recommend that only those devices that achieve a

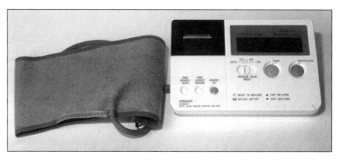

Figure 5.30 Omron HEM 705–CP monitor for self measurement of blood pressure.

Table 5.5 Automated blood pressure measuring devices for self measurement of blood pressure at the wrist, which have been subjected to validation by the BHS* and AAMI† protocols

Device	AAMI	BHS	Circumstance	Recommendation
Omron R3	Passed	NA	Intra-arterial/German	Possibly acceptable for clinical use
Omron R3	N/A	C/C	At rest; protocol violation	Unacceptable for clinical use
Boso-Mediwatch	N/A	C/C	At rest; protocol violation	Unacceptable for clinical use
Omron Rx	Failed	B/B	At rest	Acceptable for clinical use
NAIS EW 274	Failed	D/C	At rest	Unacceptable for clinical use

See notes to Table 5.2.

high grade of accuracy for both systolic and diastolic blood pressure should be recommended for clinical use.

Manufacturers are not at present obliged to guarantee the accuracy of their product, although most reputable manufacturers welcome the opportunity of having their devices evaluated independently according to a generally accepted protocol. The European Community has drawn up a directive[14-16] for all blood pressure measuring devices, which is legally binding on member states, in which it is recommended (but not obligatory) that devices should be validated independently according to a clinical protocol.

Devices for self measurement

The automated devices available for self measurement all use the oscillometric technique. There are three categories available – devices that measure blood pressure on the upper arm, the wrist, and the finger.

Finger devices

Devices that measure blood pressure at the finger are not recommended because of the inaccuracies that occur because of measurement distortion with peripheral vasoconstriction, the alteration in blood pressure the more distal the site of recording, and the effect of limb position on blood pressure.

Wrist devices

Devices that measure blood pressure at the wrist are subject to the latter two problems, and although more accurate than finger measuring devices, there are strong reservations about the correct use of these devices, especially with regard to the correct placement of the occluding cuff at heart level.

Upper arm devices

The recommendations that apply to blood pressure in general are applicable to these automated devices. Appropriate cuff sizes should be available. It may not be possible to measure blood pressure with automated devices in patients with arrhythmias, and there are some patients in whom automated measurement is not possible but for which there is no obvious reason.

User procedure

The recommendations for self measurement do not vary in principle from those that apply for blood pressure measurement in general, but there are some points in need of emphasis.[7]

Use in primary care

At present self measurement is performed mostly by patients on their own initiative using devices bought on the free market, without medical control. Self measurement should be seen by primary care physicians as offering a means of gaining further insight into blood pressure control and the effects of management strategies in motivated and informed patients who remain under medical supervision.

Devices for SBPM

- Devices for SBPM must have an EU certificate
- Devices for SBPM should be subjected to independent accuracy validation according to the AAMI or BHS protocols
- SBPM devices should provide blood pressures in both millimetres of mercury and kilopascals
- Finger measuring devices are not recommended
- Wrist measuring devices should be used with great care
- Arm measuring devices are the recommended choice
- Manufacturers should be encouraged to produce an "adjustable cuff" applicable to all adult arms
- An annual "state-of-the-market" review listing validated devices for SBPM should be published

SBPM = self blood pressure measurement

User procedure

- SBPM should be performed after a period of 5-minute rest
- SBPM should be performed with validated fully automated devices
- Use brachial artery occluding devices
- Wrist monitors are unreliable
- Device cuff must be at heart level on the arm with the highest blood pressure
- Measurement frequency
  Initial phase and the treatment period—1-week
  SBPM: 2 SBPM morning and evening
  Long term observation—minimum 1 week per quarter
- Patient diaries are unreliable
- Use printer or memory equipped devices with possibility to store or transmit
- Discard first day readings
- Use all other data to calculate the mean SBPM
- Manual device may be needed when arrhythmias are present
- SBPM should be performed under medical supervision
- Patients should be trained in SBPM and re-evaluated annually
- SBPM suited for patients motivated towards their health management
- Patients with physical or mental disabilities may be unsuited to SBPM

Frequency of measurement

The frequency of self recorded measurements may vary according to the indication and the information that is being sought. Measurements from the first day should be excluded from the statistical analysis because these may represent a period of familiarisation and anxiety with the technique, and often yield measurements that are not representative of the true blood pressure profile.[7]

Observer prejudice

The unreliability of self measured blood pressures as reported by patients themselves has been demonstrated by comparing the recorded pressures to those recorded secretly by an automatic data storage system.[7] Memory equipped devices have the potential to reduce this observer prejudice.

Training of patients

Doctors must themselves be conversant with the strengths and limitations of self measurement, and be aware of the accuracy and reliability of the equipment being used by their patients, and be able to advise them on the state of the market for automated devices.[3] Training should focus on equipment, the self measurement procedure, interpretation of results, blood pressure variability, levels of normality and the need of the calibration, and maintenance of the equipment. Towards this end nurses in primary care practices, who are most suited to training patients, may find the available CD-ROMs and the booklet of the British Hypertension Society useful for demonstration to patients anxious to know more about self measurement.[17]

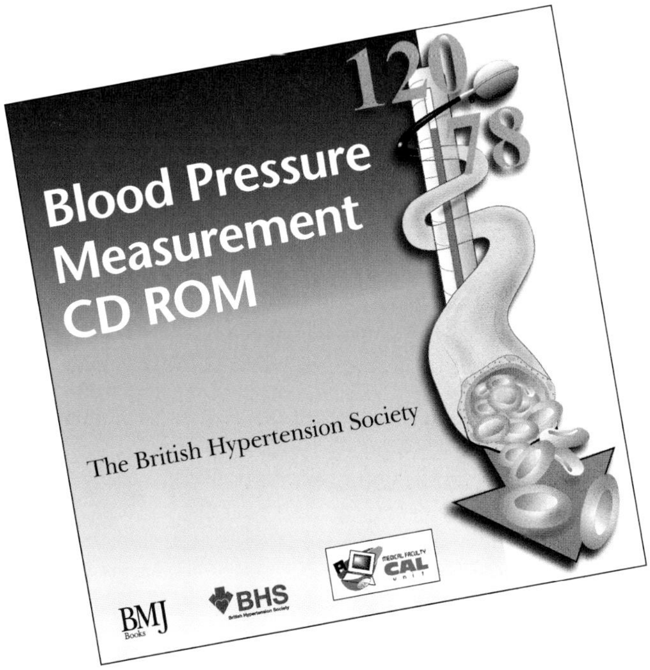

Patient requirements

Few patients are unable to perform self blood pressure measurement. The method may be advocated for hypertensive patients who would like to contribute to their own management. Self measurement may be unsuitable for patients with physical problems or mental disabilities.

Figure 5.31 Blood Pressure Measurement CD-ROM.

Diagnostic thresholds

The association between blood pressure and cardiovascular risk is continuous, without a threshold above which risk suddenly increases. However, clinical decisions must be based on diagnostic or operational thresholds. In this regard, there is an agreement that the thresholds currently applicable for conventional sphygmomanometry cannot be extrapolated to automated measurements. Different methodological approaches may be used for the determination of threshold values, the most satisfactory of which is to be able to relate blood pressure thresholds to cardiovascular outcome. However, as this data is not available for self measurement, the recommended thresholds in the box below are derived from statistical considerations in a large population database comprising some 5422 normotensive and untreated hypertensive subjects.[6-9]

Diagnostic thresholds

- Data from longitudinal studies is lacking
- Reference values are derived from statistical evaluation of databases
- 135/85 mmHg may be considered as upper limit of normality
- SBPM needs to be further evaluated in prospective outcome studies

---

Clinical indications

The clincial applications of self measurement are only beginning to become apparent as the technique becomes more widely used and scientific data is gathered; the potential uses for the technique are summarised in the box and are generally the same as for ABPM (see previous section), though the evidence for SBPM is not as strong as for ABPM.[8]

Potential clinical uses for SBPM

These applications are largely tentative and the evidence in support of the use of SBPM in these circumstances must await the outcome of ongoing studies

- White coat hypertension
- The elderly
- Pregnancy
- Hypertensive patients with diabetes mellitus
- Resistant hypertension
- Improving compliance to treatment
- Predicting prognosis
- As a guide to drug treatment

---

1 O'Brien E, Fitzgerald D. The history of blood pressure measurement. *J Hum Hypertens* 1994;**8**:73–84.

2 Laher M, O'Boyle C, Kelly J, O'Brien E, O'Malley K. Home measurement of blood pressure: training of relatives. *Ir Med J* 1981;**74**:113–14.

3 Asmar R, Zanchetti A on behalf of the Organizing Committee and participants. Guidelines for the use of self-blood pressure monitoring: a summary report of the first international consensus international conference. *J Hypertens* 2000;**18**:493–508.

4 Asmar R. Proceedings from the First International Consensus Conference on Self-Blood Pressure Measurement. *Blood Press Monitor* 2000;**5**:91–2.

5 O'Brien E, de Gaudemaria R, Bobrie G, Agabiti Rosei E, Vaisse B and the participants of the First International Consensus Conference on Self-Blood Pressure Measurement. Devices and validation. *Blood Press Monitor* 2000;**5**:93–100

6 Staessen J, Thijs L and the participants of the First International Consensus Conference on Self-Blood Pressure Measurement. Development of diagnostic thresholds for automated self-measurement of blood pressure in adults. *Blood Press Monitor* 2000;**5**:101–9.

7 Mengden T, Chamontin B, Phong Chau NG, Gamiz JLP, Chanudet X and the participants of the First International Consensus Conference on Self-Blood Pressure Measurement. User procedure for self-measurement of blood pressure. *Blood Press Monitor* 2000;**5**:111–29.

8 Herpin D, Pickering T, Stergiou G, de Leeuw, Germano G and the participants of the First International Consensus Conference on Self-Blood Pressure Measurement. Clinical applications and diagnosis. *Blood Press Monitor* 2000;**5**:131–5.

9 Imai Y, Poncelet P, Debuyzere M, Padfield PL, Van Montfrans GA and the participants of the First International Consensus Conference on Self-Blood Pressure Measurement. Prognostic significance of self-measurements of blood pressure. *Blood Press Monitor* 2000;**5**:137–43.

10 Denolle T, Waeber B, Kjeldsen S, Parati G, Wilson M, Asmar R and the participants of the First International Consensus Conference on Self-Blood Pressure Measurement. Self-measurement of blood pressure in clinical trials and therapeutic applications. *Blood Press Monitor* 2000;**5**:145–9.

11 O'Brien E, Owens P. Classic sphygmomanometry: a *fin de siecle* reappraisal. In: *Epidemiology of hypertension*. Bulpitt C, ed. *Handbook of hypertension*. Amsterdam: Elsevier, 2000:130–51.

12 American National Standard for Electronic or Automated Sphygmomanometers. ANSI/AAMI SP10-1987, *et al.* 1987, p. 25.

13 O'Brien E, Petrie J, Littler WA, de Swiet M, Padfield PL, Altman D, Bland M, Coats A, Atkins N. The British Hypertension Society Protocol for the evaluation of blood pressure measuring devices. *J Hypertens* 1993;**11**(Suppl 2):S43–S63.

14 European Standard EN 1060-1 (British Standard BSSEN 1060-1:1996). Specification for non-invasive sphygmomanometers. Part I. General requirements. 1995. European Commission for Standardisation. Brussels, 1996.

15 European Standard EN 1060-1 (British Standard BSSEN 1060-1:1996). Specification for non-invasive sphygmomanometers. Part 2. Supplementary requirements for mechanical sphygmomanometers. European Commission for Standardisation. Brussels, 1996

16 European Standard EN 1060-3 (British Standard BSSEN 1060-3:1997). Specification for non-invasive sphygmomanometers. Part 3. Supplementary requirements for electro-mechanical blood pressure measuring systems. European Commission for Standardisation. Brussels, 1997.

17 The British Hypertension Society. *Blood pressure measurement CD-ROM* London: BMJ Books, 1998.

6 Patient assessment I: clinical

No two hypertensive patients are alike and the differences between them substantially influence the thresholds for starting treatment, the choice of antihypertensive drugs, and the prognosis. The assessment of a hypertensive patient must take into account factors influencing total cardiovascular risk and not just that associated with the height of the blood pressure.

The most important aspect of the management of a patient presenting with high blood pressure is to confirm the diagnosis of hypertension. Furthermore, evaluation of associated complications or co-morbidity and the exclusion of underlying secondary causes of hypertension is part of initial patient assessment.

Multiple measurements of blood pressure over a period of time may demonstrate that blood pressure levels fall, so that a significant number of patients can no longer be regarded as hypertensive. Some patients develop high blood pressure in response to hospital or clinic attendance, the so-called "white coat effect". In some patients, blood pressures are entirely normal as soon as they leave the clinical environment. Such people are sometimes referred to as "white coat" or "office" hypertensives. Patients with white coat hypertension do not need antihypertensive therapy but need careful monitoring as they may exhibit minor vascular changes and eventually develop overt hypertension requiring treatment in the future. The use of ambulatory blood pressure monitoring (ABPM) devices has assisted in the diagnosis of this condition.

It is a fundamental error to condemn a patient to decades of medication on the basis of only one or two casual blood pressure measurements. Except for hypertensive emergencies, or those in high risk groups including those with hypertensive target organ damage, it is good practice to take multiple blood pressure readings over a few weeks or months while pursuing non-pharmacological measures before instituting drug therapy.

History

Symptoms

In the absence of any other illnesses, or the complications of hypertension, most hypertensive patients have no specific symptoms. This is reflected in the fact that many are diagnosed as an incidental finding at a routine medical examination or attendance for some other condition. There has been a common misconception that hypertensive patients complain of headaches, epistaxis, and lethargy. Although occasionally headache may be encountered, in fact even severely hypertensive individuals often have no symptoms until they present with a heart attack or a stroke. Hypertension has justly been described as the "silent killer"

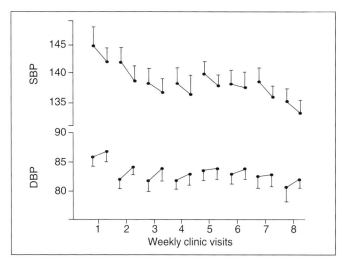

Figure 6.1 Follow up of untreated mild hypertensives demonstrating that blood pressures tend to "bottom out" at about the fourth visit. Reproduced with permission from Watson RDS, Lumb R, Young MA, Stallard TJ, Davies P, Littler WA. Variations in cuff blood pressure in untreated outpatients with mild hypertension – implications for initiating antihypertensive treatment. *J Hypertens* 1987;**5**:207–11.

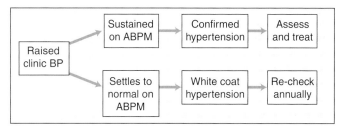

Figure 6.2 The influence of ambulatory blood pressure monitoring (ABPM) on clinical decision making.

Clinical assessment and investigation of hypertension: history	
Angina, myocardial infarction or stroke	Complications of hypertension Angina may improve when blood pressure is controlled, especially with beta-blockers
Asthma, obstructive airways disease and heart failure	Preclude the use of beta-blockers ACE inhibitors indicated in heart failure
Diabetes	ACE inhibitors are preferred
Polyuria or nocturia	Suggests renal impairment
Claudication	May be aggravated by beta-blockers. Atheromatous renal artery stenosis may be present
Gout	May be due to diuretics
Arthritis	Some non-steroidal anti-inflammatory drugs (NSAIDs) raise BP
Family history of hypertension	An important risk factor
Family history of premature death	May have been due to hypertension
Family history of diabetes	Patient may also be diabetic
Cigarette smoker	Independently causes coronary heart disease and stroke
High alcohol intake	A cause of high blood pressure
High salt intake	Important to advise restriction
Stressful lifestyle	Usually not relevant in the long term

Patient assessment I: clinical

Medical history

This may well give clues to the presence of either causes or complications of hypertension. In women, it is particularly important to inquire about their obstetric history particularly about pre-eclampsia or pregnancy related hypertension, where the risk of hypertension in later life is increased.

Family history

A family history of hypertension is found in many patients who themselves have essential hypertension. It is important to elicit whether there is a strong family history of ischaemic heart disease, stroke, or premature cardiovascular death, because this has a strong influence on the patient's own risk of cardiovascular disease. A family history of diabetes should alert the clinician to the possibility that the patient may also be diabetic. It is also important to exclude any family history of underlying disease which may cause hypertension, for example, autosomal dominant polycystic kidney disease.

Drug history

It is obviously important to enquire whether a patient is already taking antihypertensive medication and whether there has been past intolerance to any drugs. It is equally important to establish whether the patient is taking any drugs that may either cause or exacerbate the hypertension; for example, the oral contraceptive pill or carbenoxolone. Rarely liquorice or excessive use of nasal decongestants and "cold cures" may cause elevations of blood pressure. Finally, it is also important to know whether the patient is taking any medication that might interact with antihypertensive medication; for example, non-steroidal anti-inflammatory drugs which can interfere with the effects of angiotensin converting enzyme inhibitors.

Social history

The main object of a social history in the context of hypertension is to assess risk factors for both hypertension and cardiovascular disease in general. Thus it is necessary to inquire about the patient's alcohol intake, dietary habits including salt and fat consumption, and, most important of all, whether or not the patient smokes cigarettes. While there is no convincing evidence that chronic stress causes hypertension, immediate or short term stress associated with work or the home and family may cause short term rises in blood pressure. An assessment of the patient's total sense of well-being and levels of anxiety may influence the decision to treat any hypertension.

> • No two hypertensive patients are alike
> • Most have important concommitent medical problems which substantially influence the choice of treatment
> • Some are more important than the severity of the hypertension

---

Factors influencing total cardiovascular risk

Unalterable	*Treatable*
Age	Blood pressure
Gender	Serum lipids
Family history	Cigarette smoking
	Diabetes mellitus

The assessment of hypertension in women

• Prior to the menopause, the cardiovascular risk is low.
• Following the menopause, blood pressure and risks rise.
• A history of hypertension in pregnancy is probably a risk factor for later essential hypertension
• Low dose combined oral contraceptives have little effect on blood pressure and usually should not be stopped
• Hormone replacement therapy is safe in hypertensive women, but careful supervision is necessary.

Hypertension induced by drugs

• Drugs causing sodium retention: oral corticosteroids, ACTH, liquorice, carbenoxolone, indomethacin
• Drugs causing increased sympathomimetic activity: ephedrine, cold cures, monoamine oxidase inhibitors
• Direct vasoconstrictors: ergot alkaloids
• Oral contraceptives, oestrogen therapy
• Drug withdrawal: clonidine, opiates, cocaine
• Interactions with antihypertensive drugs: tricyclic antidepressants, indomethacin

---

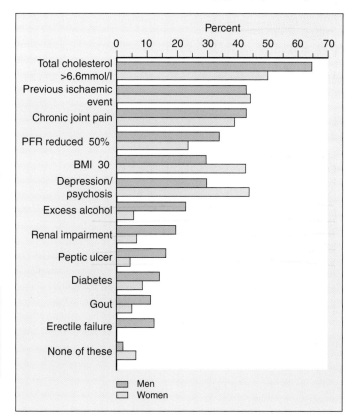

Figure 6.3 Complicating problems in 244 consecutive patients in general practice. PFR = Peak Flow Rate. Data from Hart JT. *BMJ* 1993;**306**:1337.

Physical examination

One of the most important aspects of the examination of any hypertensive patient is the measurement of height and weight. This is used to calculate the body mass index, which will allow a more accurate measure of obesity. Body weight should be checked regularly thereafter.

As with the clinical history, physical examination should include a search for the causes and the effects of hypertension, and evidence of other cardiovascular risk factors and diseases that may affect the choice of management.

General

General examination could reveal the distinctive appearance of hyper- and hypothyroidism, acromegaly or Cushing's syndrome, which are all associated with hypertension. There may be xanthelasmas associated with hyperlipidaemia, and nicotine staining of the fingers.

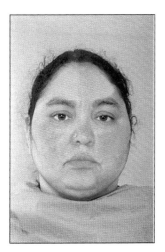

Figure 6.4 Patient with Cushing's disease and hypertension. Reproduced with permission of the patient

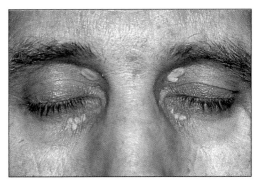

Figure 6.5 Bilateral xanthelasmas in a hypertensive patient

Body mass index (kg/m^2)	
Body mass index	*Classification*
<25	Normal
25–29	Overweight
>30	Obese

Clinical assessment and investigation of hypertension: examination	
Retinal haemorrhages and exudates with or without papilloedema	Malignant hypertension; patient should be admitted
Plethoric appearance	Consider Cushing's syndrome or high alcohol intake
Obesity	Present if BMI >25 kg/m^2
Intermittent sweating, anxiety, pallor, weight loss	Consider phaeochromocytoma
Myxoedema or thyrotoxicosis	Both give rise to hypertension
Tachycardia	Consider anxiety but exclude thyrotoxicosis
Left ventricular apical heave	Left ventricular hypertrophy, an ominous sign and treatment is urgent
Loud aortic second sound	Present in hypertension
Mitral incompetence murmur	May be due to left ventricular failure
Aortic outflow murmur	May be a flow murmur, but aortic stenosis may be present. If second sound loud may be aortic sclerosis
Pulmonary fine crepitations	Suggests heart failure. Diuretics used first, consider ACE inhibitors
Pulmonary wheezes	Avoid beta-blockers
Delayed or weak femoral pulses with precordial murmurs	Worth considering coarctation of the aorta. Measure BP in legs
Absent foot pulses	Arteriosclerosis
Abdominal mass	Autosomnal dominant polycystic kidney disease or aortic aneurysm if pulsatile
Corneal arcus or xanthelasmas	Both associated with hyperlipidaemia

Between 3 and 5 percent of all hypertensive patients have underlying causes. Most can be detected by simple clinical assessment and routine first-line investigations (see Chapter 7).

Cardiovascular and respiratory

Cardiovascular examination may reveal absent pulses or arterial bruits reflecting atheromatous disease in the femoral or carotid circulation. There may be evidence of left ventricular hypertrophy on examination of the heart, and auscultation may reveal a loud aortic second sound or cardiac murmurs. A loud systolic murmur across the chest and back, in association with delayed or weak femoral pulses and a blood pressure differential between the arms and legs, may result from a coarctation of the aorta. A high pitched early diastolic murmur suggests aortic regurgitation, which could give rise to a wide pulse pressure and apparent isolated systolic hypertension.

Examination of the chest may give evidence of obstructive airway disease, which would mean avoiding the use of beta-blockers.

Abdominal

Examination of the abdomen may reveal signs of chronic liver disease associated with high alcohol ingestion. Polycystic kidneys may be palpable on abdominal examination and a vascular bruit audible lateral to the midline might suggest renal artery stenosis.

Central nervous system

Central nervous system examination may reveal evidence of previous stroke disease.

Examination of the eyes

Ophthalmoscopy is obligatory for all patients with moderate to severe hypertension. The retinal changes can be mild or severe. The features associated with more severe hypertensive retinopathy coincides with the development of fibrinoid necrosis in the arterioles of the kidney and many other organs indicating malignant hypertension; if left untreated this is associated with an 80% two-year mortality rate. The differentiation of "accelerated" and "malignant" hypertension is not useful as the prognosis does not differ.

Ophthalmoscopy may also reveal changes of diabetic retinopathy or the characteristic appearances of retinal vein or retinal artery occlusion, which are both more common in hypertensive patients.

Retinal changes associated with hypertension

- *Mild to severe ("non-malignant hypertension")*
  Grade 1: silver wiring vessel tortuosity
  Grade 2: as above, but with arteriovenous nipping
- *Accelerated or malignant*
  Grade 3: Flame shaped retinal haemorrhages, hard exudates, cotton wool spots, macular star
  Grade 4: as above, but with papilloedema

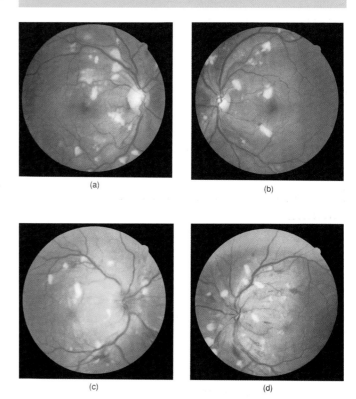

(a) (b)

(c) (d)

Figure 6.6 Retinal features in two patients with malignant phase hypertension. Upper photographs, grade III; lower photographs, grade IV retinopathy. Reproduced with permission from Lip PL, Lip GYH, Beevers DG. Hypertension illustrated: fundal changes in malignant hypertension. *J Hum Hypertens* 1997;**11**:395–6.

Further reading

- Gibbs C, Beevers DG, Lip GYH. The management of hypertensive disease in black patients. *Q J Med* 1999;**92**:187–92.

7 Patient assessment II: investigations

Each new patient requires a thorough clinical assessment, which should include a full physical examination. Tests used for the investigation of hypertensive patients can be divided into those that should be done in all newly diagnosed hypertensives and those that should be reserved for certain patients in whom the likelihood of finding a specific cause is particularly high. More detailed investigation is necessary in patients under the age of 40 years, those with resistant hypertension (that is, not responding to a combination of two or more drugs), those with severe hypertension (diastolic blood pressure >120 mmHg), and in those patients in whom clinical assessment or baseline investigations suggest that there may be an underlying cause of secondary hypertension.

Investigation for all hypertensive patients

The basic investigations should include blood biochemistry for urea and electrolytes, serum creatinine, fasting glucose and cholesterol, urinalysis for blood, protein and glucose, and an electrocardiogram (ECG).

Urinalysis

Routine stix testing of urine is the simplest but often the most revealing of the basic investigations of hypertension. Proteinuria and microscopic haematuria may both result from renal arteriolar fibrinoid necrosis in patients with malignant hypertension and also occurs in patients with non-malignant hypertension and hypertensive nephrosclerosis. They may also indicate intrinsic renal disease such as glomerulonephritis (particularly IgA nephropathy), polycystic kidney disease, or pyelonephritis. Haematuria can also occur in urological malignancy, and glycosuria may indicate coincident diabetes mellitus. In those cases where proteinuria is present, for a given level of blood pressure, the risk of death is roughly doubled.

The assessment of microproteinuria, while important in patients with diabetes mellitus, is of uncertain value in more routine hypertensive patients.

Biochemical investigations

Serum sodium concentration

This may be raised or in the high normal range in patients with primary hyperaldosteronism (Conn's syndrome). By contrast, in patients with secondary hyperaldosteronism, as occurs in chronic renal failure, serum sodium concentration can be low or low/normal. Another cause of a low serum sodium concentration is use of high doses of diuretics; occasionally profound hyponatraemia may be encountered with amiloride and hydrochlorthiazide in the combined formulation (Modiuretic).

Rationale for clinical and laboratory investigation
• Accurate diagnosis of hypertension
• Detection of other cardiovascular risk factors
• Assessment of other medical conditions which may influence choice of drug therapy
• Assessment of target organ damage
• Detection of rare underlying causes of hypertension

First line investigations	
Urine testing	
Proteinuria	Hypertensive damage diabetic nephropathy or intrinsic renal disease
Haematuria	Common in hypertensives Glomerulonephritis should be excluded Consider cystoscopy
Glycosuria	Suggests diabetes mellitus
Biochemistry	
Sodium	High in primary hyperaldosteronism (145–155 mmol/l) Usually normal or low in patients with renal hypertension (125–135 mmol/l)
Potassium	Low, due to diuretic therapy, also in chronic renal disease and primary hyperaldosteronism (1.5–3.4 mmol/l)
Creatinine	Raised in hypertensive renal damage or intrinsic renal disease. Better test than urea
Calcium	High in primary hyperparathyroidism which is associated with hypertension
Aspartate or GGT	High in patients who consume excess alcohol, with or without liver disease
Uric acid	Raised in hypertension, diuretic therapy, or heavy drinkers
Non-fasting cholesterol and HDL	Must be measured in all hypertensives to calculate cardiovascular risk
Non-fasting blood glucose	Screening for diabetes
Haematology	
Haemoglobulin	Raised in some cases of essential hypertension. Also alcohol excess. Low in chronic renal failure
Mean Cell Volume (MCV)	Raised in patients with high alcohol intake
Low platelet count	Consider connective tissue disease
ECG	Chest lead criteria for LV hypertrophy: R V5 or V6 plus SV1 >35 mm ST depression in V5 or V6 indicates "strain". Must be performed in all hypertensives
Chest X-ray	Not a reliable test for LVH. Only do if patient breathless Rib notching in coarctation of the aorta

Serum potassium concentration

This is usually low or low-normal in patients with Conn's syndrome, but the commonest cause of hypokalaemia is diuretic therapy. However if marked hypokalaemia develops in a patient receiving low dose therapy with a thiazide diuretic, an underlying diagnosis of Conn's syndrome should be considered. These drugs need to be stopped for four weeks before a true baseline serum potassium level can be established. Hyperkalaemia may be found in renal failure or with the use of some antihypertensive drugs such as the angiotensin converting enzyme (ACE) inhibitors or the potassium sparing diuretics (e.g., spironolactone or amiloride). Life-threatening hyperkalaemia has been described in patients receiving an ACE inhibitor who then opted to consume a salt substitute (Lo-Salt) which contains potassium chloride instead of sodium chloride. ACE inhibitors and potassium sparing diuretics should not be used together unless very careful monitoring of serum potassium is undertaken. However, a recent trial in patients with moderate heart failure taking ACE Inhibitors (RALES) found that low doses of spironolactone (<25 mg daily) reduced mortality by 30%.

Serum urea and creatinine concentrations

Hypertension may cause renal impairment and renal diseases cause hypertension; serum creatinine levels therefore need regular monitoring. Hypertensive patients with even a modest elevation in serum creatinine need more detailed investigation, usually in a hospital clinic.

A graph plotting the reciprocal of the serum creatinine against time may give an indication of the rate of deterioration of renal function, and hence predict the need for intervention and renal dialysis.

Serum calcium concentration

Primary hyperparathyroidism, which is associated with hypertension, causes a raised serum calcium with a low serum phosphate concentration. As with serum potassium, however, these results may be affected by the use of diuretic therapy, which modestly raises serum calcium, so these drugs need to be stopped before true baseline levels can be established.

Serum uric acid concentration

Hyperuricaemia is found in about 40% of hypertensive patients, in particular when there is renal impairment. There is also an elevation of serum uric acid with either increased alcohol ingestion or the use of thiazide diuretics. It is uncertain whether slightly raised serum uric acid levels matter in hypertensive patients without renal impairment. The evidence that serum uric acid is an independent cardiovascular risk factor is highly contentious.

Serum lipid concentrations

Although not directly related to hypertension, elevated serum cholesterol and triglyceride levels with low high density lipoprotein (HDL) cholesterol are synergistic risk factors, which need to be assessed in all hypertensive patients and treated if necessary. They may also be elevated very slightly by the use of some antihypertensive agents, such as the thiazide diuretics and non-selective beta-blockers.

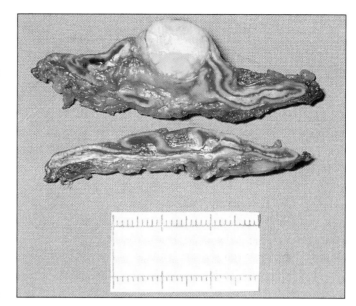

Figure 7.1 Adrenal adenoma secreting aldosterone (Conn's syndrome)

A serum potassium concentration of less than 3.5 mmol/l should be rechecked. If potassium concentration is persistently low, aldosterone excess should be considered. Remember that thiazide diuretics reduce serum potassium on average by approximately 0.2 mmol/l only

In many northern European countries, the consumption of salt-enhanced liquorice sweets is popular. Taken in excess they cause hypertension and an electrolyte profile similar to that of Conn's syndrome

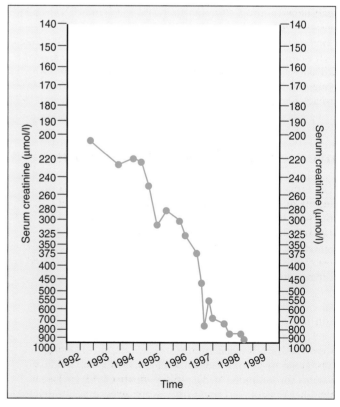

Figure 7.2 Example of a reciprocal creatinine chart in a patient with chronic renal failure. Reproduced with permission from Beevers DG, MacGregor GA. *Hypertension in practice*, Third edition. London: Martin Dunitz, 1999.

Gamma-glutamyl transferase levels

Raised gamma-glutamyl transferase levels strongly suggest an excessive alcohol intake, assuming that other intrinsic liver diseases have been excluded. There are strong associations between alcohol abuse, hypertension, and heart disease.

Haematology

Although a full blood count is a simple test, it is unlikely to provide a clear pointer to the cause or effects of hypertension. Polycythaemia may be seen in patients with chronic obstructive airways disease, Cushing's syndrome, alcohol excess and, very rarely, renal carcinoma. Anaemia in a hypertensive patient may be due to renal impairment. Plasma viscosity or ESR should only be measured if there is a suspicion of some underlying vasculitic disease.

Electrocardiography

This should be a routine investigation on all hypertensive patients, as it provides a baseline with which later changes may be compared. In addition, it may show evidence of underlying ischaemic heart disease. The most important feature of ECG in hypertension is, however, to screen for the presence of left ventricular hypertrophy (LVH), although the gold standard for assessment of LVH is echocardiography. For a given level of blood pressure, if LVH is present the mortality from heart attack, heart failure and stroke is increased three- to four-fold.

Left ventricular hypertrophy is diagnosed on the ECG when the sum of the S wave in lead V1 and the R wave in leads V5 or V6 is 35 mm or more (the Sokolow and Lyon criteria). The presence of LVH provides clear evidence of end-organ damage and a three- to four-fold excess mortality, and indicates the need for good blood pressure control. The prognosis is even worse if the "strain" pattern with ST inversion is also seen in leads V5 and V6. However, a normal ECG does not exclude the presence of LVH and there is a strong case for using echocardiography more often to diagnose cardiac enlargement.

ALL HYPERTENSIVE PATIENTS SHOULD HAVE AN ECG
• to detect LVH – a powerful risk factor
• to detect ischaemia or infarction
• if LVH absent, consider white coat hypertension
• if LVH present, ECG should be rechecked annually to monitor regression

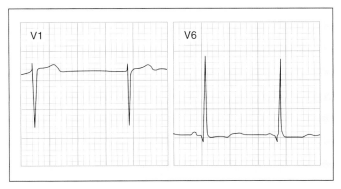

Figure 7.3 ECG demonstrating left ventricular hypertrophy and strain

Other ECG features of hypertension
• Left axis deviation
• Tall R wave in lead aVL (> 12 mm)
• Deep S wave in leads V1 and V2
• Tall R wave in leads V4 to V6
• Biphasic P wave in lead V1
• ST-T inversion leads V4 to V6 (strain)

Investigations for selected patients

More detailed investigation is usually only necessary in a minority of patients, especially the young (aged <40 years), those with severe hypertension (diastolic blood pressure >120 mmHg), resistant or uncontrolled hypertension, and suspicion of underlying disease (i.e., secondary hypertension). Most commonly it is best to refer such patients to specialised centres.

Immunology

Patients with proteinuria on dip-stick testing should be investigated to exclude vasculitis. Blood should be taken for anti-nuclear antibody (ANA) and anti-neutrophil cytoplasmic antibody (ANCA). Also urine microscopy may reveal hyaline or granular casts.

Second line investigations	
Echocardiogram	A more accurate method of assessing left ventricular size and wall thickness
Renal ultrasound	Simple non-invasive test looking for renal size, cysts, ureteric obstruction, and adrenal masses
Twenty four hour urine collections	Accurate collection is vital. Used to assess output of urinary protein, sodium, and potassium. Urine catecholes to diagnose phaeochromocytoma
24 hr ambulatory blood pressure monitoring	Expensive. Useful to assess "white coat" hypertension
Plasma renin and aldosterone	Used to diagnose primary aldosteronism
Plasma cortisol with overnight dexamethazone (1 mg) suppression test	Used to diagnose Cushing's syndrome
Thyroid function tests	Hypothyroidism is often undiagnosed

Twenty four hour urine collection

A careful 24 hour urine collection can provide valuable information in the further investigation of hypertensive patients.

- A measurement of 24 hour urinary sodium excretion may give some indication of the patient's sodium intake and provide a basis for counselling.
- For those patients whose urinalysis shows proteinuria, the 24 hour urine collection allows accurate quantification; those with more than 1 g proteinuria per 24 hours may require more specialised tests, including a renal biopsy.
- In those patients with a history suggestive of phaeochromocytoma (that is, paroxysmal or severe hypertension with sweating and palpitations), the 24 hour urine collection will allow measurement of catecholamines or their metabolites (metanephrines or vanillyl mandelic acid (VMA)).
- Cases of suspected Cushing's syndrome may be investigated with an overnight dexamethasone suppression test rather than urinary-free cortisol.
- Estimation of creatinine clearance is not necessary unless there is severe renal failure.

Radiology

Chest radiography

A chest radiograph is not necessary in most hypertensive patients. It is, however, indicated when there is clinical or ECG evidence of left ventricular hypertrophy or evidence of other heart or respiratory disease. It is best to ask the radiologist specifically to report the cardiothoracic ratio (CTR) as a measure of the amount of left ventricular hypertrophy. In aortic coarctation there may be rib notching and a figure 3 shaped descending aorta.

Echocardiography

This is primarily of use in the investigation of cardiac murmurs discovered on routine examination, although as mentioned above, echocardiography does provide the gold standard for the measurement of LVH. At present, it remains impractical to perform echocardiography on all hypertensive patients and a diagnosis of LVH is usually made on the basis of the ECG. All hypertensive patients who are breathless or develop left heart failure should undergo echocardiography to assess for left ventricular systolic (and diastolic) dysfunction.

Renal imaging

Renal ultrasonography is useful in demonstrating renal anatomy when urinalysis or serum biochemistry suggests a diagnosis of renal disease. This may demonstrate hydronephrosis, polycystic kidneys, or diminished renal size. A unilateral, smooth, small kidney may indicate renal artery stenosis that requires further investigation. In patients with intrinsic renal disease the kidneys may appear "bright" on ultrasonography. Intravenous urography is no longer used in the investigation of hypertension.

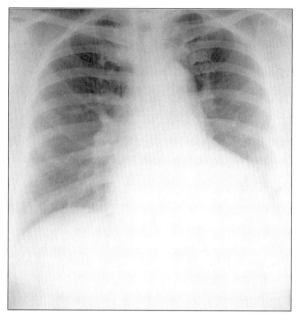

Figure 7.4 Chest radiograph of a patient with malignant hypertension, showing cardiomegaly

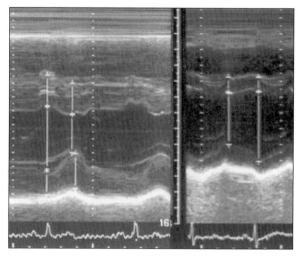

Figure 7.5 Two-dimensional and M-mode echocardiograms showing: *left*, severe left ventricular hypertrophy with marked thickening of the intraventricular septum and posterior wall; *right*, normal echocardiogram

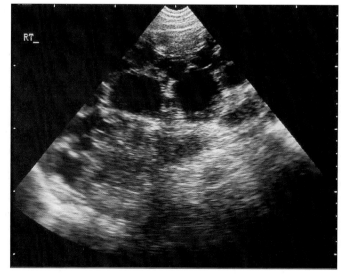

Figure 7.6 Ultrasound showing polycystic kidney

Renal angiography

This is the "gold standard" for the diagnosis of renal artery stenosis, although the procedure does carry some risk. It may be indicated in patients with severe resistant hypertension even when other evidence of renal artery stenosis is lacking. More recently, magnetic resonance (MR) renal angiography has been introduced and this may become the investigation of choice to diagnose renal artery stenosis.

Computed tomography or magnetic resonance imaging (MRI)

Either of these tests can be used for the localisation of phaeochromocytomas or adrenal tumours causing aldosterone excess. Small tumours may, however, still be missed and computed tomography may not pick up generalised adrenal hyperplasia.

Radioisotope imaging

Standard renal radioisotope imaging now has little to offer in the investigation of hypertension. The captopril renogram may, however, give additional evidence in support of the diagnosis of renal artery stenosis. In this test, radioisotope imaging of the kidneys is performed before and after administration of a dose of captopril. The isotope image of the kidney on the affected side is reduced following the captopril dose. Radioisotope imaging may also be useful in the localisation of phaeochromocytomas using scans with meta-iodobenzylguanidene (MIBG scan). Iodo-cholesterol radioisotope imaging has little value in the diagnosis of aldosterone-secreting adrenal adenomas.

Plasma hormone concentrations

These are necessary to confirm the diagnosis of an endocrine cause of secondary hypertension. Conn's syndrome results in a raised plasma aldosterone concentration with suppressed plasma renin activity. By contrast, secondary hyperaldosteronism gives rise to raised plasma aldosterone concentrations together with raised plasma renin activity. It is important that these tests are measured with the patient both fasting and supine, preferably before rising in the morning, and then with the patient ambulant 2 hours later. More recently there has been a trend to look for abnormalities of the renin-aldosterone ratio rather than for simply high plasma aldosterone.

Investigations for Cushing's syndrome should be conducted in all patients with a "Cushingoid" appearance with a plethoric round face, hirsutites, central obesity with red abdominal striae but without obesity in the arms and legs. Random cortisol assays can be misleading and there is no substitute for an overnight dexamethasone (1 mg) suppression test. The differentiation between adrenocorticotropic hormone (ACTH) secreting tumours and adrenal tumours secreting cortisol requires specialised endocrinological tests and computed tomography scans.

Acromegaly may be suspected from the clinical appearance of the patient; its investigation is through glucose tolerance testing with growth hormone levels and computed tomography scans of the pituitary fossa.

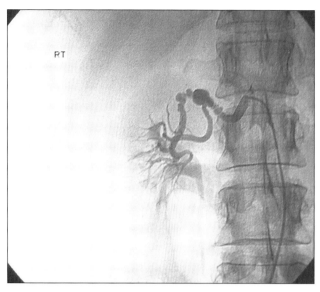

Figure 7.7 Fibromuscular dysplasia on renal angiography

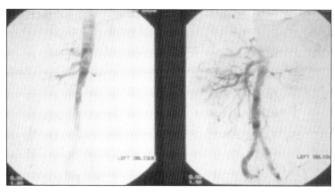

Figure 7.8 Angiogram showing left atheromatous renal artery stenosis and extensive aortic atheroma

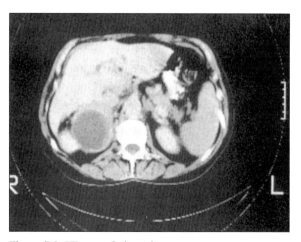

Figure 7.9 CT scan of phaeochromocytoma

Hormones measured in some hypertensive patients	
• Aldosterone	raised in Conn's syndrome and renal hypertension
• Renin	low in Conn's syndrome; high in renal disease
• Catecholamines	raised in phaeochromocytoma
• Cortisol	Cushing's syndrome
• Thyroxine and TSH	Hypo- and hyper-thyroidism
• Parathormone	Hyperparathyroidism
• Female sex hormones	HRT

Primary hyperparathyroidism is diagnosed by the presence of a normal or raised parathyroid hormone concentration in the presence of raised serum calcium concentration.

The diagnosis of phaeochromocytoma is normally made from a combination of the patient's symptoms and the 24 hour urinary catecholamine analysis. This technique will, however, miss the diagnosis in a few patients and plasma noradrenaline concentrations may then be more specific in those patients where there is a high index of suspicion.

Further reading

- Berglund G, Anderson O, Wilhelmsen L. Prevalence of primary and secondary hypertension: studies in a random population sample. *BMJ* 1997;**2**:554–6.
- Bravo EL, Tarazi RC, Dustan HP *et al.* The changing clinical spectrum of primary aldosteronism. *Am J Med* 1983;**74**:641–51.
- McInnes GT, Semple PF. Hypertension: investigation, assessment and diagnosis. *Br Med Bull* 1994;**50**:443–59.
- Ross EJ, Griffith DNW. The clinical presentation of phaeochromocytoma. *Q J Med* 1989;**71**:485–6.
- Rostand SG, Brown G, Kirk KA, Rutsky EA, Dustan HP. Renal insufficiency in treated essential hypertension. *New Engl J Med* 1989;**320**:684–8.

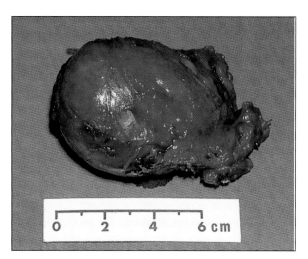

Figure 7.10 Phaeochromocytoma removed from a patient with severe hypertension.

8 Treatment of uncomplicated hypertension: non-pharmacological treatment

The management of the hypertensive patient requires confirmation of the diagnosis, assessment of the patient for underlying cause(s) and target organ damage, and initiation of appropriate therapy. Effective management of hypertension requires the identification of those at highest cardiovascular risk and the adoption of multifactorial intervention, targeting not only blood pressure levels, but also associated cardiovascular risk factors. The 1999 British Hypertension Society guidelines recommend that cardiovascular risk should be calculated based on the Framingham risk function, in keeping with the Joint British Societies' recommendations on cardiovascular prevention, to estimate 10-year coronary heart disease risk. Colour charts and computer programs are available for risk estimation (see Appendix).

Non-pharmacological treatment

Before a patient begins to take any antihypertensive medication, it is appropriate to attempt non-pharmacological measures to lower blood pressure. These measures should also be used in all patients who are receiving antihypertensive drug therapy.

A number of lifestyle modifications, such as weight reduction, salt and alcohol restriction and regular exercise, do produce significant falls in blood pressure and can also improve other cardiovascular risk factors. These may obviate the need for pharmacological treatment, or at least have an additive effect when combined with drug therapy. In some patients, stringent non-pharmacological measures may occasionally allow reduction in or cessation of drug therapy. The 1999 guidelines of the British Hypertension Society and the US Joint National Committee urge that non-pharmacological measures should be used in all hypertensive patients.

Obesity

There is a strong association between obesity and hypertension. Several studies have shown that a reduction in systolic and diastolic pressures occurs with weight loss: a reduction in weight of 3 kg produces a fall in blood pressure of about 7/4 mmHg; a reduction of 12 kg gives a fall of 21/13 mmHg. Every attempt should be made to encourage obese patients to diet so that their weight falls to within the norm for their height and build. Available evidence suggests that the results achieved with the help of dieticians are better than those achieved by medical staff alone.

Salt

Dietary sodium intake in most people eating a Western diet is grossly in excess of that required for health. As suggested by the Intersalt study, there is a clear relationship between dietary salt intake and blood pressure, and people who consume less salt have a smaller rise in blood pressure with advancing age. Salt restriction to about 100 mmol/day has been shown to produce a significant reduction in blood

Non-pharmacological blood pressure reduction

1 *Definitely effective*
   a   avoidance and control of obesity
   b   restriction of salt intake
   c   moderation of alcohol intake
   d   increase potassium intake (fruit and vegetables)
   e   low fat diet

2 *Ineffective*
   a   raised calcium intake
   b   relaxation therapy, yoga, and biofeedback
   c   vitamins, folic acid, traditional herbal remedies.

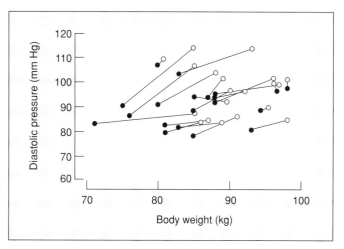

Figure 8.1 Relationship of weight change and blood pressure change: from the Framingham study. Reproduced with permission from Staessen J, Fagard R, Amery A. The relationship between body weight and blood pressure. *J Human Hypertens* 1988;**2**:207–17.

It may help to tell the patients that for every pound in weight they lose, the blood pressure will fall by about 1 mmHg on average

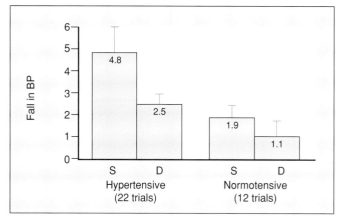

Figure 8.2 Overview of trials of salt restriction. Reproduced with permission from Cutler JA, Follmann D, Allender PS. Randomized trials of sodium reduction: an overview. *Am J Clin Nutr* 1997;**65**(Suppl):643s–51s.

pressure in several randomised placebo controlled studies. Suitable dietary salt restriction can be achieved by not adding salt at the dining table and avoiding notoriously salty foods such as hamburgers, sausages, and salty bacon. Processed foods often contain vast quantities of salt and should therefore be avoided as much as possible. Many supermarkets now are reducing the salt content of their own brand processed and convenience foods, and patients should be advised accordingly. Most patients who convert to a low salt diet find that within a few weeks they prefer this and actively dislike the salt in foods they once routinely consumed.

Some patients use salt substitutes containing potassium chloride; while these may be beneficial, there is a risk of life threatening hyperkalaemia when these salt substitutes are combined with angiotensin converting enzyme (ACE) inhibitors or potassium sparing diuretics.

There is some evidence that patients of African Caribbean origin are more sensitive to a given dietary salt load. However, it is now also becoming clear that restriction of salt in their diet has a greater blood pressure lowering effect. For this reason particular efforts should be made to counsel these patients.

There is also some evidence that older hypertensive patients are more salt sensitive than younger patients.

Salt restriction in people without hypertension also lowers blood pressure modestly, with some evidence that those with a family history of hypertension are more salt sensitive. It is to be hoped that a national reduction of dietary salt intake can be achieved, and this may reduce the prevalence of hypertension in the population at large.

Potassium

While increasing potassium intake with potassium tablets is emphatically not recommended, there is good evidence that increasing potassium intake with a diet high in fruit and vegetables does lower blood pressure and may also independently prevent strokes.

Dairy products

Lowering the dietary intake of saturated fats may bring about a fall in blood pressure, but there remains some uncertainty. A recent study, the DASH (Dietary Approaches to Stop Hypertension) trial, has demonstrated that a low fat diet, together with an increase in fruit and vegetables, can significantly lower blood pressure more than simply an increase in fruit and vegetables alone. A low fat diet also has other benefits in the prevention of coronary heart disease.

Summary of dietary recommendations

The simplest advice to give to patients is that they should try to eat more fresh foods with plenty of vegetables and avoid processed or convenience foods.

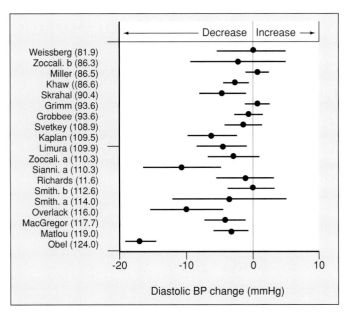

Figure 8.3 Overview of clinical trials of potassium supplementation on blood pressure. Figures in brackets represent average baseline diastolic blood pressures. Reproduced from Cappuccio FP, MacGregor GA. Does potassium supplementation lower blood pressure? A meta-analysis of published trials. *J Hypertens* 1991;**9**:465–73.

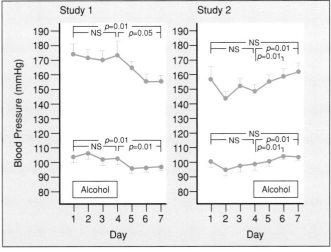

Figure 8.4 Effects of potassium supplementation in different studies in order of severity of initial blood pressure. Figures in parentheses represent the mean arterial pressure on entry to the study. Adapted with permission from Potter JF, Beevers DG. Pressor effect of alcohol in hypertension. *Lancet* 1984;**i**:119–22.

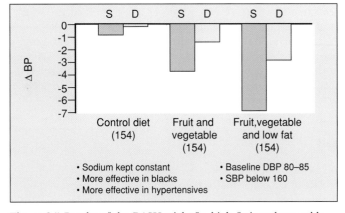

Figure 8.5 Results of the DASH trial of a high fruit and vegetable and low fat diet. Data from Appel LJ, Moore TS, Obarzanek E *et al.* A clinical trial of the effects of dietary patterns on blood pressure. *New Engl J Med* 1997;**336**:1117–24.

Alcohol

The association between alcohol intake and hypertension is well documented in both population and clinical studies. An alcohol intake of around 80 g alcohol/day (equivalent to 4 pints of beer) has been shown to raise blood pressure, particularly in hypertensive patients. Blood pressure falls soon after drinking is stopped or reduced and remains low in those who continue to abstain. Where relevant, hypertensive patients should be encouraged to reduce their alcohol intake to an average of 21 units/week in men and 14 units/week in women (1 unit being equivalent to one glass of wine or sherry, one tot of spirits, or half a pint of beer).

Exercise

Epidemiological studies on exercise and blood pressure are difficult to assess because they can easily be confounded by differences in diet and lifestyle. There are, however, some reliable studies now available, which show that a graduated exercise programme is associated with clinically useful reductions in blood pressure in hypertensive patients. Indeed, 30–45 minutes of modest aerobic exercise, such as a brisk walk or a swim three times a week, produces a modest fall in blood pressure. Newly diagnosed, obese, hypertensive patients with ischaemic heart disease should not suddenly take up jogging, but a sensibly administered increase in physical exercise is beneficial in such patients.

Smoking

The most effective lifestyle measure to reduce overall cardiovascular risk is smoking cessation, and every effort should be made to encourage hypertensive smokers to quit. Nicotine replacement should be made available where appropriate. Smoking cessation will not, however, reduce blood pressure and, if weight gain occurs, there may even be a small rise.

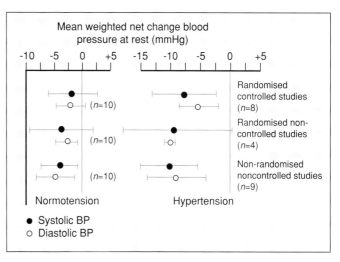

Figure 8.6 Overview analysis of studies of the change in blood pressure resulting from physical training. Reproduced with permission from Fagard RH. The role of exercise in blood pressure control: supportive evidence. *J Hypertens* 1995;**13**:1223–7.

Further reading

- Alderman MH. Non-pharmacological treatment of hypertension. *Lancet* 1994;**344**:307–11.
- Beilin LJ. Epitaph to essential hypertension – a preventable disorder of known aetiology. *J Hypertens* 1988;**6**:85–94.
- Joint National Committee on Detection, Evaluation and Treatment of High Blood Pressure. Non pharmacological approaches to the control of high blood pressure. *Hypertension* 1986;**8**:444–67.
- Ramsay LE, Yeo WW, Chadwick IG, Jackson PR. Non-pharmacological therapy of hypertension. *Br Med Bull* 1994;**50**:494–508.

9 Treatment of uncomplicated hypertension: pharmacological treatment

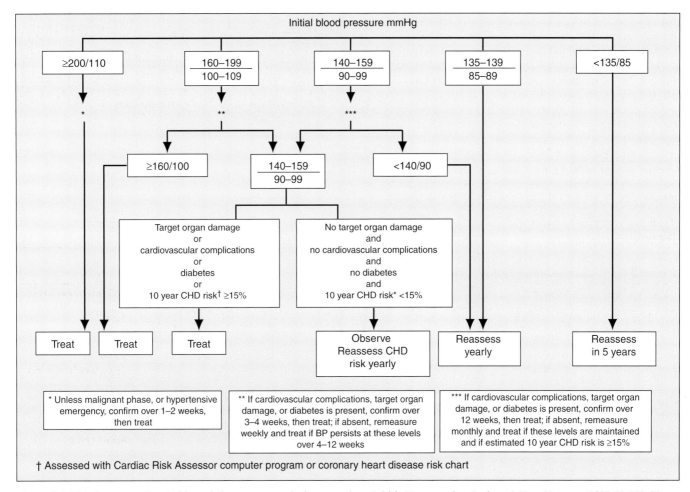

Figure 9.1 Blood pressure thresholds and drug treatment in hypertension. British Hypertension Society. *J Hum Hypertens* 1999;**13**:569–92.

When to use drugs

As mentioned previously, the most universally accepted definition of hypertension is "That level of blood pressure above which investigation and treatment do more good than harm". With this in mind, guidelines for treatment have been devised taking into consideration the available data on the risks of hypertension and the benefits of its treatment.

The current British and American guidelines suggest that we should use drug treatment in those patients under 80 years of age with a diastolic blood pressure of >100 mmHg. This threshold should be reduced to 90 and 99 mmHg when there is evidence of end-organ damage or coexisting risk factors. In addition, the guidelines recommend that we should treat patients (particularly those aged over 60) with systolic blood pressures >160 mmHg even if the diastolic blood pressures are below 90 mmHg. Again this threshold should be reduced to 140 mmHg in diabetics and patients with target organ damage. The aim of treatment should be to reduce diastolic blood pressure to below 90 mmHg, and systolic blood pressure to below 140 mmHg. The guidelines also urge that blood pressures should be measured on four separate occasions before taking the decision to prescribe antihypertensive drugs.

Which drugs to use?

The traditional approach to the drug treatment of hypertension has been "stepped care", that is, starting treatment with a thiazide or beta-blocker and progressing, if necessary, to a combination of the two with the addition of a vasodilator if needed. The introduction of calcium channel blockers and angiotensin converting enzyme (ACE) inhibitors and a resurgence in the popularity of alpha-blockers have seen a move away from this approach.

Most clinicians would now favour "tailored care" of the patient's needs, which means that any of the above mentioned types of drugs could be used as first line therapy, taking into account the patient's individual characteristics in terms of concomitant disease, and cardiovascular risk factors, as well as social and economic considerations in deciding on the most appropriate therapy. Furthermore, the beta-blockers and thiazides are no longer the only drugs that have been proved to reduce mortality and morbidity for hypertension. However, many patients with hypertension fall into a number of special groups where there are either compelling indications for a particular agent from randomised controlled trials or good reasons to believe a particular agent will have favourable effects on a co-morbid condition.

There have been a great many clinical trials comparing different antihypertensive drugs, but there is only one reliable trial that has compared the efficacy and tolerability of all five first line drug groups – the TOMHS (Treatment Of Mild Hypertension Study) study. The outcome of the study showed that all the major drug groups are efficacious in the treatment of mild hypertension (including the thiazides) and that the incidence of side effects and tolerability differs from one drug group to another. Nevertheless, we need more information whether the newer agents (calcium antagonists and ACE inhibitors) are better than the older agents (thiazides and beta-blockers), and ongoing trials such as ALLHAT (Antihypertensive and Lipid Lowering Heart Attack Trial) and ASCOT (Anglo-Scandinavian Cardiac Outcomes Trial) will answer this question.

Both the British and American guideline committees took the view that, bearing in mind hypertension is particularly a problem in older patients, the thiazide diuretics were the optimal first line drugs. If for some reason the thiazides

The decision to start antihypertensive treatment must be based on:

1 Assessment of the patient's total cardiovascular risk, taking into account age, gender, familial history, smoking and cholesterol as well as the blood pressure.
2 Awareness that if NIDDM is present, the risk is increased to the same level as a non-diabetic heart attack survivor.
3 Evidence from reliable clinical trials that blood pressure lowering is worthwhile.
4 Evidence that non-pharmacological manouvres have been complied with.
5 Detailed explanation to the patient of the risks of hypertension and the benefits of treatment.

Table 9.1 Compelling and possible indications and contraindications for the major classes of antihypertensive drugs. Reproduced with permission from British Hypertension Society. *J Hum Hypertens* 1999;**13**:569–92.

| | Indication | | Contraindication | |
Class of drug	Compelling	Possible	Possible	Compelling
Alpha-blockers	Prostatism	Dyslipidaemia	Postural hypotension	Urinary incontinence
ACE inhibitors	Heart failure Left ventricular dysfunction Type I diabetic nephropathy	Chronic renal disease* Type II diabetic nephropathy	Renal impairment* Peripheral vascular disease†	Pregnancy
Angiotensin II receptor antagonists	Cough induced by ACE inhibitor‡	Heart failure Intolerance of other antihypertensive drugs	Peripheral vascular disease†	Pregnancy Renovascular disease
Beta-blockers	Myocardial infarction Angina	Heart failure§	Heart failure§ Dyslipidaemia Peripheral vascular disease	Asthma or chronic obstructive pulmonary disease Heart block
Calcium antagonists (dihydropyridine)	Isolated systolic hypertension in elderly patients	Angina Elderly patients	—	—
Calcium antagonists (rate limiting)	Angina	Myocardial infarction	Combination with beta-blockade	Heart block Heart failure
Thiazides	Elderly patients	—	Dyslipidaemia	Gout

*Angiotensin converting enzyme (ACE) inhibitors may be beneficial in chronic renal failure but should be used with caution. Close supervision and specialist advice are needed when there is established and significant renal impairment
†Caution with ACE inhibitors and angiotensin II receptor antagonists in peripheral vascular disease because of association with renovascular disease
‡If ACE inhibitor indicated
§Beta-blockers may worsen heart failure, but in specialist hands may be used to treat heart failure

Table 9.2 Checklist of common or important side effects with different classes of antihypertensive drugs

Common side effect	Diuretic	Beta-blocker	ACE inhibitor	Angiotensin receptor antagonist	Calcium antagonist	Alpha-blocker
Headache	–	–	–	–	+	–
Flushing	–	–	–	–	+	–
Dyspnoea	–	+	–	–	–	–
Lethargy	–	+	–	–	–	–
Impotence	+	+	–	–	–	–
Cough	–	–	+	–	–	–
Gout	+	–	–	–	–	–
Oedema	–	–	–	–	+	–
Postural hypotension	–	–	–	–	–	+
Cold hands and feet	–	+	–	–	–	–
Stress incontinence	–	–	–	–	–	+
Angioedema	–	–	+	+	–	–
Constipation	–	–	–	–	+	–

cannot be used, because of side effects, then calcium channel blockers can be used, as they were shown to prevent vascular events in the SYST-Eur trial. The beta-blockers have to a lesser extent been validated in preventing vascular events and so could also be considered as first line therapy, although they tend to be less effective in elderly hypertensives and African Caribbean subjects.

A 10 year coronary heart disease (CHD) risk of 15% is equivalent to a total cardiovascular disease (CVD) risk of 20% (i.e., including strokes and heart failure)

Diuretics

The thiazide diuretics remain the mainstay of treatment of hypertension. They are cheap, easy to use, and can be given once daily. They are particularly suitable for elderly and African Caribbean patients. Conversely, however, they tend to be less effective in younger white patients. There is little to choose between the various thiazides, although it seems prudent to use agents such as hydrochlorothiazide and bendrofluazide that have been proved to be effective at low doses in clinical trials. Newer agents, such as indapamide, may have fewer metabolic side effects. The thiazides are one of the classes of antihypertensives that have been extensively tested in large long term outcome trials. In the early trials, thiazides reduced the incidence of stroke by the 40% expected from epidemiological studies, although the reduction in coronary heart disease was disappointing, perhaps because of the adverse metabolic effects of the large doses used. More recent trials using lower doses have demonstrated impressive reductions in both strokes and coronary heart disease, especially in the elderly. Diuretic drugs are particularly useful in combination with the beta-blockers and ACE inhibitors.

These drugs are absorbed from the gut and excreted through the kidney. They act on the distal renal tubules, thereby increasing sodium, potassium and water excretion. However they also have some direct arteriolar vasodilating properties. These two mechanisms combine to produce a gradual decline in blood pressure (over four weeks), which is equal to that produced by other agents. The dose-response curve with respect to blood pressure is flat, so that increasing the dose beyond a certain threshold has little further antihypertensive effect but causes more metabolic abnormalities.

Loop diuretics such as frusemide are less potent antihypertensive agents as they produce a brisk but short lived diuresis and are thus unsuitable as first line agents for hypertension. These agents are only indicated either when there is concomitant cardiac or renal failure, or in resistant hypertensive patients receiving ACE inhibitors. Metolazone is a powerful thiazide-like diuretic that is also used in resistant hypertension. Spironolactone is a specific aldosterone antagonist, with a particular role in primary hyperaldosteronism (Conn's syndrome) and heart failure.

Adverse effects

The main concerns about the thiazide diuretics are the metabolic side effects, but with low doses these are uncommon. Predictably thiazide diuretics cause a small fall in serum potassium due to renal potassium excretion. Hypokalaemia is more common in patients treated with the thiazide than the loop diuretics, and the risks of mild hypokalaemia in hypertension are uncertain, but it may potentially result in ventricular arrhythmias and cause adverse effects in patients on digoxin or drugs that prolong the QT interval on the ECG (e.g. Class I antiarrhythmics, tricyclic antidepressants,

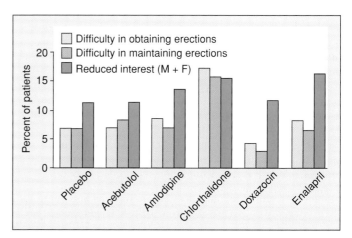

Figure 9.2 BP drugs and sexual function in the TOMHS study

Metabolic side effects of bendrofluazide 2.5 mg. Carlsen JE, Køber L, Torp-Pederson OC, Johansen P. Relation between dose of bendrofluazide, antihypertensive effects and adverse biochemical effects. *BMJ* 1990;**300**: 975–8

	Baseline	*2.5 months*	*% change*
Potassium	4.25	4.05	–4.7
Urate	0.32	0.35	9.0
Creatinine	81.5	84.0	3.1
Glucose	4.7	4.9	2.9
Cholesterol	5.86	5.86	0

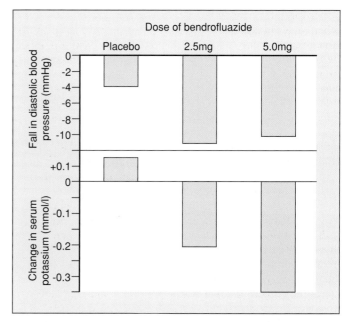

Figure 9.3 Effects of placebo and bendrofluazide, 2.5 or 5.0 mg daily, on diastolic blood pressure and serum potassium. Adapted with permission from Carlsen *et al. BMJ* 1990;**300**:975–8

antihistamines). However if hypokalaemia occurs with a low dose of a thiazide diuretic a diagnosis of underlying aldosterone excess should be considered. Acute gout is another common side effect of thiazides even in low doses. Hyperuricaemia can be present in about 30% of hypertensives, but is a poor predictor of acute gout. Impotence may occasionally be a problem. Thiazides can increase serum LDL-cholesterol and triglyceride levels, but this is much less of a problem with modern low doses. They also may impair glucose tolerance and increase insulin resistance, but the provocation of frank diabetes mellitus is rare. Although thiazides probably should be avoided as first line drugs in non-insulin dependent diabetics and those with hyperlipidaemia, there should be no anxiety about adding them in where necessary to achieve better blood pressure control. Rarer side effects include nausea, headache, rashes, photosensitivity, and blood dyscrasias.

The metabolic side effects of the thiazides continue to increase with escalating doses, so lower doses are now recommended (e.g., bendrofluazide 2.5 mg or hydrochlorothiazide 25 mg once daily) than have been prescribed in the past. Hypokalaemia can be avoided through prescription of low doses of thiazides; it is also less common in patients with a restricted salt intake. If, however, hypokalaemia is persistent, the diagnosis of Conn's syndrome (primary hyperaldosteronism) should be considered.

Beta-blockers

The beta-blockers inhibit the action of catecholamines on beta-adrenoreceptors. Some block both beta$_1$-receptors (heart rate and contractility) and beta$_2$-receptors (vascular and bronchial smooth muscle), whereas others mainly block beta$_1$-receptors and are therefore relatively cardioselective. Their major effect is to slow the heart rate and reduce the force of contraction of the heart. Beta-blockers also cause some reduction in renin release and central sympathetic tone. They tend to be less effective in the elderly and in black hypertensives.

Used carefully they are effective and safe, and are well absorbed from the gastrointestinal tract. Some are metabolised in the liver and some excreted renally, so the dose must be reduced in patients with renal failure; others are excreted via either route. Beta-blockers are thought to lower blood pressure through a reduction in cardiac output, but they also suppress the release of renin; some may also have a central effect on the vasomotor centre. As with thiazide diuretics, beta-blockers show a flat dose-response curve for blood pressure. There is little value in increasing the dose above that recommended, although higher doses may be tried in black patients who are less responsive to beta-blockers. Beta-blockers also have antianginal properties so are useful in hypertensive patients with angina. In addition they have secondary preventive properties in postmyocardial infarction patients. Recent data suggests a beneficial effect on patients with heart failure.

Beta adrenergic receptor blockers may be subdivided according to their ancillary properties. For example, beta$_1$ or cardioselective agents (such as atenolol, metoprolol, and bisoprolol) have less action on beta$_2$-adrenoreceptors in the bronchi and peripheral vessels. This reduces (but does not abolish) beta$_2$-receptor mediated side effects. Lipid soluble agents such as propranolol and metoprolol cross the blood-brain barrier more readily and cause more "central" side effects of lethargy, sleep disturbance, and vivid dreams. Some beta-blockers, such as pindolol, have intrinsic sympathomimetic activity, and therefore cause less bradycardia

---

Diuretics in the year 2000

- The thiazide group of diuretics should remain the drugs of first choice in older patients
- The dose of thiazide diuretics should be as low as possible
- The metabolic side effects of the thiazides can be minimised if low doses are used
- The best drugs to add in to bendrofluozide are the ACE inhibitors or the beta blockers

---

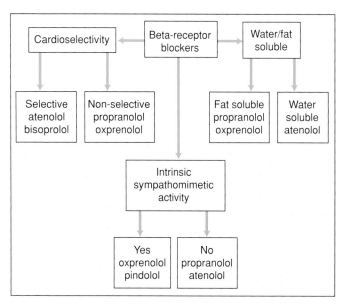

Figure 9.4 Non-cardioselective beta-blockers tend to cause more bronchospasm. Those with intrinsic sympathomimetic activity cause less bradycardia on cold extremities. Fat-soluble beta-blockers cause more vivid dreams and sleep disturbance whilst water soluble drugs may be retained in renal failure.

Meta-analysis of effects of Beta-blockers on mortality and admissions to hospital in chronic heart failure

No. of trials (total no. of patients)	% inpatients receiving placebo	% inpatients on active treatment	Risk reduction (%)	P value
18 (3023)	24.6	15.8	38	<0.001

Beta blockers in the year 2000

- When first introduced, the beta blockers were a major breakthrough in the treatment of hypertension
- Their use is declining slightly because the newer drugs have fewer side effects
- Beta blockers must be used in certain situations
  a) Heart attack survivors
  b) Angina pectoris
  c) Stable left ventricular failure
- In hypertension their role is more commonly as an add in drug but in low dosage (e.g. atenolol 25–50 mg daily)
- It is possible that the newer beta blockers nebivolol, celiprolol, and bisoprolol have fewer side effects
- Propranolol should no longer be used for hypertension

and possibly fewer problems with cold extremities than other beta-blockers. Labetolol and carvedilol have both alpha-blocking and beta$_1$-blocking properties, leading to a reduction in peripheral vascular resistance as well as slowing the heart rate, but they are not more effective than the conventional beta-blockers.

Contrary to early expectations, the beta-blockers were not better than the thiazides at preventing the vascular complications of hypertension. They were also slightly less effective at lowering blood pressure, especially in older patients.

Adverse effects and contraindications

Most of the side effects of beta-blockers are predictable from their mode of action. Thus, beta-blockers are contraindicated in patients with a history of wheeze or in those with heart block on their ECG. Sinus bradycardia is common and is not a reason to stop beta-blockers unless the patient is symptomatic or the heart rate falls below 40/minute. Lipid soluble agents can cause central nervous system side effects of insomnia, nightmares, and fatigue. Exercise capacity may be reduced and most patients experience generalised low grade lethargy.

Like the diuretics, non-selective beta-blockers can worsen glucose intolerance and hyperlipidaemia. In diabetics prone to hypoglycaemia, beta-blockers may theoretically reduce the awareness of low blood glucose. Given the array of side effects that may adversely affect a patient's quality of life, it is questionable whether beta-blockers are really suitable as first line drugs for mild uncomplicated hypertension.

Calcium channel blockers

The calcium channel blockers are a chemically heterogeneous group that acts through inhibition of the transfer of calcium ions across cell membranes, reducing intracellular calcium and smooth muscle contraction leading to vasodilation. Calcium channel blockers differ in their affinity for cardiac conducting tissues (slowing atrioventricular nodal conduction), cardiac muscle (reducing contractility), and vascular smooth muscle (peripheral vasodilatation). All are well absorbed from the gastrointestinal tract and undergo first pass metabolism in the liver.

The dihydropyridines, such as nifedipine and amlodipine, have little effect on the atrioventricular node but are potent vasodilators, and also have some mild diuretic effects. The older calcium antagonists such as nifedipine in capsule form have short half-lives and may cause rapid vasodilation, a reflex tachycardia and catecholamine surges, and may aggravate myocardial ischaemia. Longer acting agents such as amlodipine or slow release preparations of nifedipine partially overcome these problems.

Verapamil is a useful antiarrhythmic drug with some vasodilatory action. It slows atrioventricular node conduction and reduces myocardial contractility. Diltiazem has some effect on both cardiac conduction and vascular smooth muscle.

In the mid-1990s, a series of pharmacosurveillance case control studies suggested that the short acting dihydropyridine calcium antagonists (such as nifedipine capsules) actually increased the risk of heart attacks, haemorrhage, cancer, and suicide. Recently the SYST-Eur trial demonstrated that treatment with the short acting dihydropyridine calcium antagonist, nitrendipine, reduced strokes and heart attacks, without an increase in conditions previously attributed to the calcium antagonists.

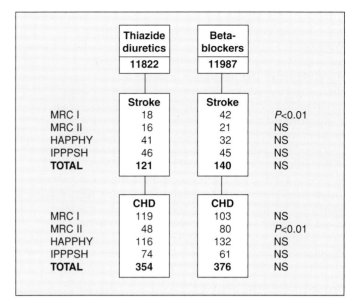

Figure 9.5 Beta-blockers versus thiazides – hard endpoint trials in hypertension. Reproduced with permission from Beevers DG. Beta-blockers for hypertension: time to call a halt. *J Hum Hypertens* 1998;**12**:807–10

Three types of calcium channel blocker

- Dihydropyridines (which include nifedipine, nicardipine, and amlodipine)
- Verapamil
- Diltiazem

A comparison of specific calcium channel blockers

	Verapamil	Nifedipine	Diltiazem
Systemic arteriodilatation	2	3	1
Hypotensive effect	2	3	1–2
Coronary arteriodilatation	1	3	1
Reduced cardiac contractility	2	1	1
Impaired sinus and AV node function	3	0	3
Antiarrhythmic effect	3	0	3
Antianginal effect	2–3	2–3	2–3

0 = No discernible action; 3 = Potent effect

Calcium channel blockers in the year 2000

- These drugs have now been validated in long term outcome studies (NORDIL, INSIGHT, SYST-Eur)
- Short acting nifedipine must not be used in unstable angina or post myocardial infarct patients
- Suspicions that calcium channel blockers are unsafe are not born out by the randomised trials listed above
- In older patients these drugs are the best alternative to the thiazide diuretics

Adverse effects

The most troublesome side effects of the calcium antagonists are ankle oedema, headache, flushing, and palpitation, especially with short acting dihydropyridines. These side effects are dose related and may occasionally improve with continued use and can be offset by combining a calcium antagonist with a beta-blocker. The ankle oedema is thought to result from a direct effect of these drugs on capillary permeability and is not responsive to diuretics.

Verapamil and diltiazem are contraindicated in patients with heart block and should not be used in patients taking digoxin or the beta-blockers. They also increase plasma concentrations of digoxin. Verapamil has fewer of the side effects of the peripheral vasodilatatory type, but may cause troublesome constipation. Verapamil and diltiazem as well as short acting dihydropyridines are best avoided in heart failure.

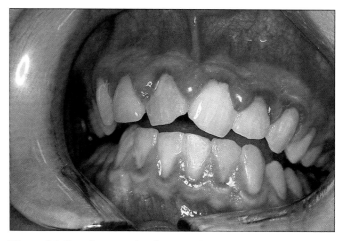

Figure 9.6 Gum hypertrophy due to amlodipine.

Angiotensin converting enzyme inhibitors

The role of the renin-angiotensin-aldosterone system in the control of blood pressure is described in Chapter 4 on the pathophysiology of hypertension. The ACE inhibitors block this system and cause a reduction in blood pressure through a reduction in peripheral vascular resistance and, to a lesser extent, through prevention of the renal absorption of sodium by aldosterone. Their effects probably result through inhibition of both systemic and local tissue renin systems. ACE inhibitors also reduce the breakdown of the vasodilator bradykinin, which may enhance their action but is responsible for their most troublesome side effect of cough. Furthermore, ACE inhibitors may improve endothelial function and reduce central adrenergic tone. They also have beneficial effects on renal haemodynamics, reducing postglomerular efferent arteriolar constriction and intraglomerular pressure, resulting in reduction of proteinuria and rate of decline in renal function in patients with various forms of nephropathy.

These drugs show little difference in their actions, except for the duration of action and route of excretion. Other agents, such as fosinopril, have the advantage of hepatic as well as renal excretion and are therefore (theoretically, at least) less likely to accumulate in renal failure. Perindopril, ramipril and trandolapril are agents with long half-lives, thus providing good 24–hour antihypertensive coverage. They are all well tolerated in uncomplicated hypertension but should be used with care in elderly people, patients with renal impairment (because renal function may deteriorate), and patients taking diuretics (to avoid precipitous falls in blood pressure). Treatment should be introduced in low doses and increased gradually over the course of a few weeks.

There is useful synergism between the ACE inhibitors and the diuretics or calcium antagonists. The ACE inhibitors are particularly useful in diabetic hypertensives, where they may be renoprotective, slowing the progression of diabetic nephropathy; furthermore, these agents have shown some benefits in delaying diabetic retinopathy and even neuropathy. In patients at cardiovascular risk, the recent HOPE study (see box) demonstrates a benefit of ACE inhibitors independent of their blood pressure lowering effect. However, the ACE inhibitors tend to be less effective as antihypertensive agents in black/African Caribbean hypertensives and the elderly, due to their low renin state. Nevertheless, this relative ineffectiveness can be overcome by using high doses or adding a diuretic or calcium channel blocker.

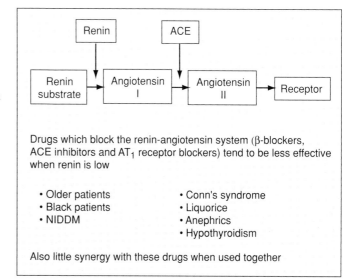

Figure 9.7 The limitations of drugs which block the renin-angiotensin system. NIDDM = non-insulin-dependent diabetes mellitus

HOPE (Heart Outcomes Prevention Evaluation Study)
n = 9297 "high risk" subjects (*New Engl J Med* 2000;**342**:145–53)

- Ramipril reduces the rate of death, MI, stroke, revascularisation, cardiac arrest, heart failure, complications related to diabetes and new cases of diabetes in a broad spectrum of high-risk patients
- Only a small part of the benefit attributed to reduction in BP as reduction in BP was extremely small (3/2 mmHg)
- The magnitude of the benefit at least as large as that observed with other proven secondary prevention measures, e.g. beta-blockers, aspirin and statins

Treating 1000 patients with ramipril for four years prevents about 150 events in approximately 70 patients

Adverse effects

Cough due to the inhibition of bradykinin breakdown is the most common side effect of ACE inhibitors, occurring in 10% of men and 20% of women, particularly if they are non-smokers. The far more serious, but rare, side effect of the ACE inhibitors is acute angioedema, which occurs in about 0.1–0.2%, and is twice as common in black patients. Dramatic deteriorations in renal function can occur in patients with bilateral renal artery stenosis. Serum urea and creatinine should therefore be checked before and at a few weeks after starting an ACE inhibitor. This should not prevent the use of ACE inhibitors in those with other forms of renal disease in whom they are often agents of first choice, in view of data showing that ACE inhibitors slow the progression of both diabetic and non-diabetic nephropathy.

Because of their effect of reducing aldosterone and thus potassium excretion, the ACE inhibitors can cause hyperkalaemia. First dose hypotension is probably an overstated side effect, but large doses of short acting captopril can cause sudden falls in blood pressure, especially in those with volume depletion such as heart failure patients on large doses of diuretics. Rarer side effects include rash, taste disturbance, blood dyscrasias, and a symptom complex including fever and vasculitis.

Alpha-receptor antagonists

The alpha$_1$-adrenoreceptor blockers produce vasodilatation by blocking the action of norepinephrine (noradrenaline) at postsynaptic alpha$_1$-receptors in both arteries and veins, resulting in a fall in peripheral resistance without a compensatory rise in cardiac output. The prototype alpha$_1$-blocker prazosin is short acting and tends to produce precipitate falls in blood pressure, but the longer acting doxazosin combines the advantage of a more gentle reduction in blood pressure with once daily dosing.

Until recently, these drugs have been out of favour for the treatment of essential hypertension. With the introduction of once daily preparations (doxazosin and terazosin), however, they have experienced a resurgence in popularity. Theoretically, there are no absolute contraindications to this group of drugs. They may cause dizziness and postural hypotension, and symptoms associated with vasodilatation. Alpha$_1$-adrenoreceptor blockers produce comparable reductions in blood pressure to other first line antihypertensive drugs. They seem to be particularly useful as a third drug, producing good falls in blood pressure where two agents combined have failed. In contrast to the beta-blockers and diuretics, alpha$_1$-adrenoreceptor blockers actually produce modest improvements in serum lipids and glucose tolerance, but whether this translates into improved outcomes is not known because of the paucity of long term outcome data with these agents. Of concern is the termination of the doxazosin arm of ALLHAT due to an increase in heart failure and stroke (see box)

Side effects

The main side effect is postural hypotension with the shorter acting agents. In women alpha$_1$-adrenoreceptor blockers may cause urinary incontinence but in men they may improve the symptoms of benign prostatic hypertrophy. Like most antihypertensive drugs alpha$_1$-adrenoreceptor blockers can cause headache and fatigue.

The ACE-inhibitor-induced cough may annoy the patient's spouse particularly at night

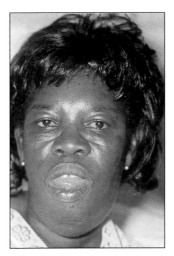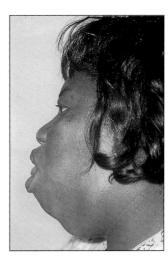

Figure 9.8 Acute angioedema due to enalapril in an African Caribbean patient (published with permission from the patient).

ACE Inhibitors in the year 2000

- There is, as yet, no evidence that the ACE inhbitors are superior to other drugs in routine essential hypertension
- There is evidence that the ACE inhibitors are the best drugs to reduce LVH
- ACE inhibitors are the drugs of first choice in IDDM and NIDDM
- ACE inhibitors preserve renal function in hypertensives with mild to moderate renal failure

Antihypertensive and Lipid-Lowering Treatment to Prevent Heart Attack Trial (ALLHAT) – Results of Alpha blockers

- Doxazosin arm stopped in January 2000
- Doxazosin arm (n=9067) and the chlorthalidone group (n=15268) similar for baseline characteristics
- At 4 years, 86% of patients on chlorthalidone were still taking the drug (vs 75% in the doxazosin arm)
- Mean systolic BP was 135 mmHg in the chlorthalidone group vs 137 mmHg in the doxazosin arm

Relative risk (RR) *doxazosin vs chlorthalidone*
- CHD   1.03 (95% CI 0.9–1.17)
- Combined CVD   1.25 (95% CI 1.17–1.33; P<0.001)
- CHF   2.04 (95% CI 1.79–2.32)
- stroke   1.19 (95% CI 1.01–1.4; P=0.04)

Alpha blockers in the year 2000

In the light of the ALLHAT findings, these drugs should be resent for use as 2nd or 3rd line therapy where now pressure is uncontrolled

Angiotensin receptor blockers

Like the ACE inhibitors these drugs act on the renin-angiotensin system blocking the action of the angiotensin II at its peripheral (AT1) receptors. As they do not inhibit the breakdown of bradykinin they do not cause cough but may lack the additional physiological benefits of rises in bradykinin levels.

It therefore appears that they have all the advantages of ACE inhibitors but none of the disadvantages. There is synergism of antihypertensive effect by addition of a thiazide diuretic. There is also some evidence that they may regress left ventricular hypertrophy and improve proteinuria. Ongoing studies are examining their role in heart failure due to systolic dysfunction. The ELITE trial showed no significant difference in all cause mortality between captopril (15.9%) and Losartan (17.7%), but better tolerability with the latter.

Adverse effects

The main advantage of the angiotensin II antagonists is their apparent lack of side effects. Like the ACE inhibitors, they may cause hyperkalaemia, renal impairment, and hypotension, but otherwise they are almost as well tolerated as placebo. Nevertheless, cases of angioedema have been reported with some of these agents.

Other drugs

Central alpha-adrenoceptor and imidazoline agonists

These drugs stimulate central $alpha_2$-adrenoceptors, resulting in a decrease in central sympathetic tone. This leads to a fall in both cardiac output and peripheral vascular resistance. Examples of such drugs include methyldopa and clonidine. Nevertheless, they cause sedation, a dry mouth, and fluid retention. Methyldopa can also cause autoimmune hepatic derangement and haemolytic anaemia. However, methyldopa is safe in the hypertensive pregnant woman. A new centrally acting drug, moxonidine, acts on central imidazoline receptors and is hoped to have the beneficial effects of centrally acting drugs without their side effects.

Reserpine also has centrally mediated antihypertensive properties but in high doses causes depression and even suicide. However it is very cheap and in combination with a thiazide diuretic (also cheap) low doses are effective. While hardly used in Western countries, this combination can be used, with care, in developing countries where financial considerations are paramount.

Direct vasodilators

These agents act directly to relax vascular smooth muscle, thereby reducing peripheral vascular resistance. The resulting activation of the sympathetic nervous system means that they can only successfully be used in combination with beta-blockers. Examples include hydralazine, where the main side effect is a lupus-like syndrome, and minoxidil, which causes hair growth, a side effect welcomed by many middle aged men but not by their female counterparts! Hydralazine may be used for resistant heart failure in combination with nitrates, although its use for essential hypertension is much less widespread.

Figure 9.9 Angiotensin II receptors and their blockade

	Blocked by:
Angiotensin II → AT₁ receptor → Vasoconstrictor	Losartan, Valsartan, Candesartan, Irbesartan, Eprosartan, Telmisartan
Angiotensin II → AT₂ receptor → Vascular growth and remodelling	

Angiotensin receptor blockers in the year 2000

- Angiotensin receptor blockers do not block the AT₂ receptor, and because they raise plasma angiotensin levels, the receptor is stimulated
- The role of the AT₂ receptor is uncertain but may be important in fetal growth
- Thus angiotensin receptors are absolutely contraindicated in pregnancy
- Almost no side effects are encountered
- The results of long term outcome studies will become available in 2002–2004

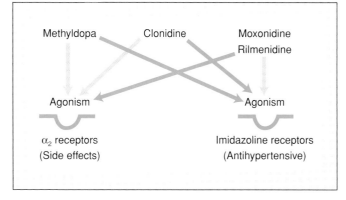

Figure 9.10 Central antihypertensive agents (SIRA – Selective Imidazoline Receptor Agonists)

Hydralazine can cause a lupus-like reaction with joint pains and renal vasculitis. Its use can only be justified in hypertension where all else fails or in heart failure where ACE inhibitors cannot be used or do not alone control symptoms

Combination therapy

Firstly it must be accepted by doctors, nurses and patients that with the new targets for blood pressure reduction, only about 25% of all hypertensive patients will achieve satisfactory blood pressure control with only one drug. Most patients will require double or triple drug therapy.

If a particular antihypertensive drug is proving ineffective, then the addition of a second drug may be the next appropriate step. As an alternative, a switch to a drug from a different group may be worthwhile. Either of these steps is preferable to increasing the dose of the original drug to its maximum, because most side effects are dose related.

In choosing which drugs to use in combination, it is important to appreciate their modes of action and to choose a combination of drugs that complement each other. For example, the addition of a diuretic to a beta-blocker or ACE inhibitor is a logical step. Diuretics exert their effect on blood pressure by a reduction in the circulation volume, which is partially offset by an increase in plasma renin activity. If the renin-angiotensin system is subsequently blocked, this will produce a synergistic antihypertensive effect. By contrast, the combination of diuretics and calcium channel blockers is not a logical one and, in practice, produces little extra reduction in blood pressure.

In order to aid the clinician in sensible prescribing we have developed the "Birmingham Hypertension Square" for add-in drugs in the management of hypertension. The clinician should opt to approach the square from any corner, with first-line drugs chosen logically. The optimal second line agents are immediately adjacent and indicated by the arrows.

The choice of the third agent is less certain and there is little hard data. It is probable that there are no firm rules, and one could "go on round the square" or add in an alpha-blocker or a centrally acting agent.

In the HOT study only 25% of patients achieved adequte BP control with monotherapy
Most hypertensive patients need two or more drugs

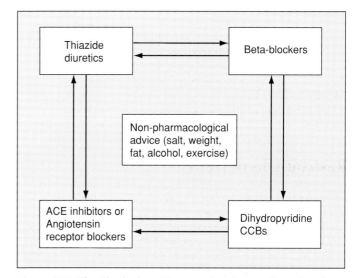

Figure 9.11 The Birmingham Hypertension Square. Reproduced with permission from Lip GYH, Beevers M, Beevers DG. *J Hum Hypertens* 1998;**12**:761–3.

Aspirin

In the HOT (Hypertension Optimal Treatment) trial, aspirin 75 mg daily in treated hypertensive patients aged 50 years or more reduced cardiovascular events by 15% and myocardial infarction by 36%, but had no effect on strokes or total fatal events. There were in fact only 46 fewer heart attacks, but 57 more episodes of bleeding. In the Thrombosis Prevention Trial of aspirin 75 mg daily for primary prevention (26% had treated hypertension) showed a 16% reduction in all cardiovascular events, a 20% reduction in myocardial infarction, and no effect on fatal events. The HOT trial studied well controlled hypertensives, and in the Thrombosis Prevention Trial aspirin was withheld when blood pressure was above 170/100 mmHg

Hypertension must therefore be well controlled (<150/90 mmHg) before starting aspirin treatment for primary prevention of cardiovascular disease in hypertensive subjects. For example, those who developed cerebral haemorrhage in the Thrombosis Prevention Trial had significantly higher systolic blood pressures before the event (158 mmHg, vs 135 mmHg in those with no stroke).

Patients with an estimated 10-year CHD risk of >15% will have their cardiovascular risk reduced by 25% using antihypertensive treatment. The addition of aspirin further reduces major cardiovascular events by 15%, giving a NNT (number needed to treat) for 5 years of about 90 for one cardiovascular complication and 60 for one myocardial infarction prevented by aspirin.

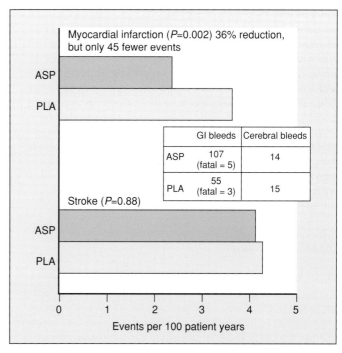

Figure 9.12 HOT (Hypertension Optimal Treatment) trial results: aspirin (ASP) 75 mg vs placebo (PLA). Data from Hansson L, Zanchetti A, Caruthers SG *et al*. Effects of intensive blood pressure lowering and low dose aspirin in patients with hypertension: principal results of the Hypertension Optimal Treatment randomised trial. *Lancet* 1998;**351**:1755–62.

Lipid lowering

The value of lowering plasma lipid levels with a statin is firmly established in all hypertensive and diabetic patients who have recovered from a myocardial infarction. The threshold for starting therapy in such patients is 5.0 mmol/l.

In hypertensive patients with no complications the situation is less clear, and both the ASCOT and ALLHAT trials are investigating lipid lowering in patients with cholesterol levels between 5.0 and 6.5 mmol/l. Above 6.5 mmol/l cholesterol lowering drugs should probably be given.

In the meantime the British Hypertension Society guidelines recommend that uncomplicated hypertensive patients should receive lipid lowering drugs if their 10-year coronary risk exceeds 30%. To identify these patients, the clinician should refer to the colour charts and the Joint British Societies Cardiac Risk Assessor computer program (see appendix A). Thus it is mandatory to measure plasma lipids (including HDL-cholesterol) in all hypertensive patients. It should be noted that an unexpected finding in the trials of HMG coenzyme A inhibitors (statins) was also a reduction in strokes (by approximately a third) as well as heart attacks.

Resistant hypertension

If the diastolic blood pressure is still over 100 mmHg after triple drug treatment, consideration should be given to whether the patient is actually complying, as drug regimes can often be simplified to improve compliance. It is also worthwhile to double check that there is no underlying renal or adrenal cause for the hypertension. These patients are probably best referred to specialist hospital clinics. When essential hypertension is genuinely resistant to treatment, the substitution of frusemide or metolazone for the thiazide diuretic may further reduce the blood pressure.

Another approach is to use minoxidil, which has a direct effect on arterioles by causing vasodilatation, although it does not dilate veins. Side effects are common, so this drug is reserved for patients with genuinely severe and resistant hypertension. Fluid retention and tachycardia mean that minoxidil must be used together with a loop diuretic and a beta-blocker. Hypertrichosis occurs after about three weeks of treatment; it is reversible but may be cosmetically unacceptable to women.

Some patients require four or even five different antihypertensive drugs to control their blood pressure. Under these circumstances, long acting, once daily drugs are preferable, so that they may still only need to take four or five tablets once daily.

Based on the 1999 British Hypertension Society Guidelines, aspirin 75 mg daily is recommended for hypertensive patients who have no contraindication to aspirin; in one of the following categories:

- *Secondary prevention* – cardiovascular complications (myocardial infarction, angina, non-haemorrhagic stroke, peripheral vascular disease, or atherosclerotic renovascular disease).
- *Primary prevention* – with blood pressure controlled to <150/90 mmHg and either: (a) age >50 years and target organ damage (e.g., left ventricular hypertrophy, renal impairment, or proteinuria); or (b) a 10-year CHD risk >15%; or (c) type 2 diabetes mellitus.

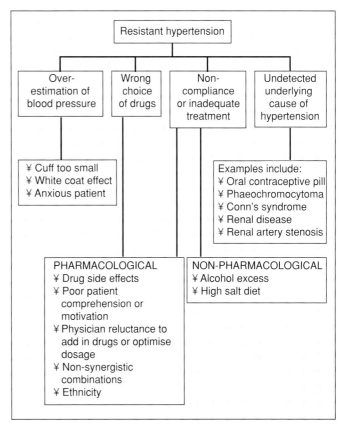

Figure 9.13 Strategies for the management of resistant hypertension

- Severe hypertension under good control carries a good prognosis
- Milder hypertension under poor control carries a less good prognosis
- The target is 140/80 mmHg and lower in diabetic patients

Treatment of uncomplicated hypertension: pharmacological treatment

Antihypertensive drugs – the Birmingham list

Examples	Mode of action	Indications	Contraindications/side effects
Thiazide diuretics:			
Bendrofluazide Hydrochlorothiazide	Diuretic and vasodilator, very slow onset	Inexpensive. Use lowest dose possible Suitable for the elderly or added to ACE inhibitors or beta-blockers	May cause hypokalaemia, a rise in lipids and glucose intolerance Impotence
Beta-blockers:			
Atenolol Metoprolol Bisoprolol	Reduces cardiac output Suppresses renin release Slows pulse rate Anti-anginal action	Used in patients with angina, myocardial infarction, stable heart failure and young, nervous, patients	Do not give to asthmatics or patients with peripheral vascular disease May cause vivid dreams, fatigue and lethargy
Angiotensin converting enzyme (ACE) inhibitors:			
Lisinopril Enalapril Captopril Ramipril	Inhibits conversion of angiotensin I to angiotensin II	Where beta-blockers contraindicated or not tolerated Indicated in heart failure, diabetes and renal impairment	Care if renal impairment or widespread atheroma 10–20% of patients develop dry cough Enalapril or captopril are given twice daily Angioedema (1 in 4000)
Calcium channel blockers:			
Amlodipine Nifedipine LA Verapamil Diltiazem	Vasodilator Useful for emergencies (nifedipine)	Older patients Black patients Patients with peripheral vascular disease angina. Useful with ACE inhibitors and beta-blockers	Flushing, headache, ankle swelling, gum hypertrophy Verapamil should not be used with beta-blockers Avoid nifedipine retard in patients with CHD
Alpha-blockers:			
Doxazosin Terazosin	Blocks alpha-receptors on arterioles	May help sexual function in men and relieve prostatism	Safe, causes dizziness and stress incontinence in women
Angiotensin receptor antagonists:			
Losartan Valsartan Candesartan	Blocks angiotensin receptors in arterioles	Best used where ACE inhibitors cause side effects	Almost no side effects Care in patients with renal impairment
Central alpha agonists and imidazoline receptor agonists:			
Methyldopa Moxonidine	Reduces cerebral sympathetic activity	Pregnancy (methyldopa only)	Depression and sedation

Further reading

- Guidelines Subcommittee. 1999 World Health Organisation – International Society of Hypertension guidelines for the management of hypertension. *J Hypertens* 1999;**11**:905–18.
- Neaton JD, Grimm RH, Prineas RJ *et al*. Treatment of Mild Hypertension Study: Final results. *JAMA* 1993;**270**:713–24.
- The Sixth Report of the Joint National Committee on prevention, detection, evaluation and treatment of high blood pressure (JNC-V1). *Arch Intern Med* 1997;**157**:2413–46.

10 Hypertension in special cases

The treatment of hypertension has now moved away from the concept of a rigid stepped care approach towards a view of tailoring treatment to the patient's individual needs. This chapter looks at the management of hypertension in particular groups of patients, especially those with pre-existing cardiovascular damage and those with other important concomitant medical conditions that influence the choice of treatment.

Ethnic groups

Hypertension is particularly common in African Caribbean black populations, with a prevalence as high as 50% over the age of 40 years in the United States. Although hypertension is more common, it remains uncertain whether any particular level of blood pressure is associated with a worse prognosis than in whites. Although things may be changing, black hypertensives have lower risk of coronary heart disease but conversely a higher risk of stroke, renal failure, and left ventricular failure. The blood pressure is particularly more sensitive to dietary salt restriction, and in mild hypertensive patients without evidence of target organ damage, a low salt diet may occasionally be sufficient to control blood pressure. There is some evidence that black patients are more sensitive to the harmful effects of salt excess but also the beneficial effects of salt restriction compared to white patients, and advice on self restriction is particularly important. There is little convincing evidence that black patients consume more salt than whites but they may well consume less potassium in the form of fruit and vegetables.

It is now well documented that black people tend to have different responses to antihypertensive medication from those of white and Asian people, and it is thought that this is related to their low plasma renin and angiotensin levels. Black people are known to respond poorly to beta-blockers and angiotensin converting enzyme (ACE) inhibitors, although treatment with the thiazide diuretics and calcium channel blockers is effective. However, these patients may respond to ACE inhibition or beta-blockade when these drugs are given in high doses, or in combination with drugs that activate the renin-angiotensin system, such as the diuretics or calcium channel blockers. In resistant hypertension a combination of diuretic, calcium antagonist, ACE inhibitor and/or alpha-blocker is particularly effective.

South Asians (from the Indian subcontinent) in Britain also have a high prevalence of hypertension, are commonly insulin resistant, and have a high prevalence of type 2 diabetes. They are at an increased risk of stroke and a very high risk of coronary heart disease. The limited evidence available suggests that the responses to drug treatment of hypertension in South Asian patients is generally similar to that in white Europeans. Important points in management are the particular emphasis on glucose tolerance, lipids, and the increased coronary risk. The thiazide diuretics, which can worsen glucose intolerance, should therefore be used with caution. Clear advice is needed to reduce fat (particularly saturated fats as in ghee) and refined sugar intake and to increase regular physical exercise. Good control of blood pressure is particularly important in patients with diabetes, and aspirin and/or statin treatment may be indicated for those at high risk of coronary heart disease.

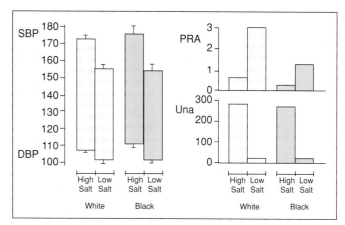

Figure 10.1 The effects of dietary salt restriction on blood pressure and plasma renin activity (PRA) in African Caribbean and white hypertensive patients. He FJ, Markaadu ND, Sagnella GA, MacGregor GA. Importance of the renin system in determining blood pressure fall with salt restriction in black and white hypertensives. *Hypertension* 1998;**32**:820–4.

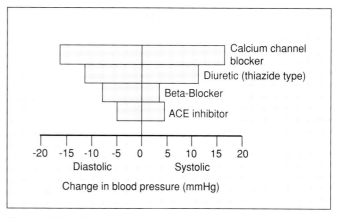

Figure 10.2 Antihypertensive drug response in black patients. Reproduced with permission from Hall WD. Pathophysiology of hypertensives in blacks. *Am J Hypertens* 1990;**3**:3665–715.

Ethnic differences and treatment

Ethnic group		
Black	High incidence of stroke	Respond poorly to beta-blockers and ACE inhibitors
		More sensitive to salt
Asian	High risk of CHD	No clear evidence of differences in drug response
	High risk of diabetes mellitus	

There is little information on hypertension in people of Chinese origin. In some groups, salt intake is very high. It is possible that ACE inhibitor induced cough is more common than in caucasians.

Malignant hypertension

Malignant hypertension is diagnosed by the presence of advanced hypertensive retinopathy (haemorrhages, cotton wool spots, exudates with or without papilloedema) in the presence of a diastolic blood pressure of over 120 mmHg. It is more common in black people and in smokers. The prognosis for untreated malignant hypertension is appalling and worse than that for many cancers, with 88% dead in two years. Even when treated, a high proportion of patients develop complications such as stroke or renal failure. Again this is particularly a problem in black patients, although this may be a reflection of more severe hypertension and greater renal impairment at first presentation, rather than a true effect of ethnicity. The presence of renal impairment at presentation (serum creatinine >300 μmol/l) and the quality of blood pressure control at follow up are the main determinants of prognosis.

It is important that malignant hypertension is investigated thoroughly to detect underlying renal, renovascular and adrenal diseases. Vascular complications are found more frequently than in non-malignant hypertension (although malignant hypertension secondary to Conn's syndrome is extremely rare). Most patients who have malignant hypertension do not have an obvious underlying cause, although many have evidence of renal damage (e.g., proteinuria). There is uncertainty about whether this results from underlying renal disease (e.g., IgA nephropathy) or arteriolar fibrinoid necrosis caused by the malignant hypertension.

The treatment of malignant hypertension should be prompt, although it is unnecessary, and indeed unwise, to treat these patients with parenteral antihypertensive drugs. Precipitous falls in blood pressure from very high levels are dangerous and can lead to the development of acute stroke. Perhaps the only indications for use of parenteral antihypertensive drugs are in the very rare patients with hypertensive encephalopathy or where the patient has severe hypertension, that is diastolic blood pressure >130 mmHg, but is unable to take oral medication due to impaired level of consciousness.

The initial aim of treatment in malignant hypertension is to lower the diastolic blood pressure by 20–25% in the first 48 hours and aim for a target blood pressure of around 100 mmHg, using combination therapy if necessary. The maximum initial fall in blood pressure should not exceed 25% of the presenting value in order to avoid underperfusion of the brain, heart, and kidneys. All patients with malignant hypertension should be admitted to hospital and the blood pressure should be monitored four hourly and lowered gradually over the first few days with oral therapy only. A gradual reduction of blood pressure will allow adaptation of disordered cerebral blood flow autoregulation and avoid target organ ischaemia. The first line oral antihypertensive agent is either a short acting calcium antagonist (e.g., nifedipine 10–20 mg) or a beta-blocker (e.g., atenolol 25–50 mg). Doses can be repeated or increased at intervals of 6–12 hours, to bring about a gradual reduction in blood pressure.

The use of sublingual nifedipine capsules is obsolete and dangerous, especially since the drug is not absorbed from the buccal mucosa, and the erratic absorption after crushing nifedipine capsules can lead to precipitous falls in blood pressure and can cause strokes or heart attacks. An alternative

> Malignant hypertension
>
> - If untreated, 88% dead in 2 years
> - If long term, BP control good, 5-year survival is 80%
> - Dangerous to normalise BP too quickly
> - Parenteral drugs must not be used unless severe LVF or encephalopathy
> - Retinopathy "heals" in 2–3 months

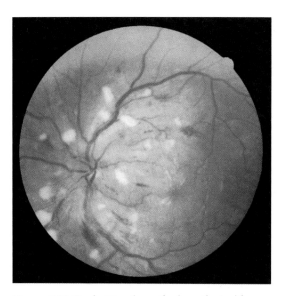

Figure 10.3 Grade IV retinopathy in patient with malignant phase hypertension

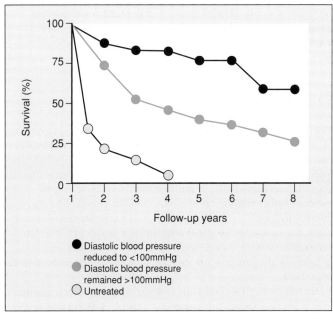

Figure 10.4 Survival rates for untreated and treated malignant hypertension. Reproduced with permission from Beevers DG, MacGregor GA. *Hypertension in practice*, Third edition. London: Martin Dunitz, 1999.

drug is atenolol which may be used in small doses, increasing if necessary, or in combination with a calcium antagonist. Nevertheless, beta-blockers should only be used if there is no asthma or heart failure and there is no suggestion that the patient has a phaeochromocytoma. Beta-blockade without an alpha-blocker may give rise to a hypertensive crisis in the patient with phaeochromocytoma. ACE inhibitors may produce rapid and dangerous falls in blood pressure, particularly in patients with renovascular disease, which may be undiagnosed in the acute situation, and are therefore not recommended as first line therapy. Diuretics are inadvisable as these patients are often mildly fluid depleted, presumably secondary to pressure related diuresis and activation of the renin-angiotensin system. They should be given only if there is evidence of heart failure or fluid overload.

Hypertension following a stroke

Severe hypertension post stroke is a risk factor for further stokes and long term treatment is worthwhile. It is unclear whether the treatment of mild hypertension post stroke is of benefit, especially because immediately after a stroke, there is a breakdown of cerebral blood flow autoregulation so that rapid falls in blood pressure can cause a reduction in cerebral perfusion and an extension of the stroke. Nevertheless most clinicians would prescribe antihypertensive drugs.

What therefore is the role of antihypertensive medication pre, during and post stroke? This can be summarised as follows:

- *"Pre"*: many randomised controlled trials have demonstrated that it is of benefit to have hypertension treated aggressively to <140/85 mmHg.
- *"During"*: it is detrimental to have hypertension treated aggressively. If the blood pressure persistently exceeds 180/110 mmHg, then nifedipine 10–20 mg tablets or atenolol 25 mg should be prescribed. In patients already receiving antihypertensive medication, this is best withdrawn and only reinstated at a later stage.
- *"Post"*: this question still remains unanswered in mild hypertension, even though the patients are at high risk.

Antihypertensive therapy is best withheld until the patient is ambulant. If it can be proved that the stroke was the result of a cerebral infarct, then low dose aspirin (150 mg) is mandatory once the blood pressure is controlled.

Left ventricular hypertrophy

The presence of left ventricular hypertrophy (LVH) is evidence of target organ damage. However LVH is also an independent risk factor for cardiovascular mortality and, where present, for a given level of blood pressure, the mortality is three to four times higher (Fig 10.7). Patients with LVH have a higher incidence of sudden cardiac death, arrhythmias (ventricular arrhythmias and atrial fibrillation), heart failure, stroke, coronary artery disease, and peripheral vascular disease. In patients with atrial fibrillation, the presence of concomitant hypertension is additive to the risk of stroke, especially if LVH is present.

It has been shown that most drugs in current use as first line therapy bring about a reduction in LVH associated with a reduction in blood pressure. Three recent meta-analyses have, however, strongly suggested that the ACE inhibitors are more effective than other drugs at reducing LVH (Fig 10.8). It is believed that this may be because angiotensin II has a growth

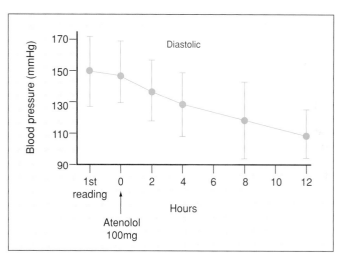

Figure 10.5 The immediate effects of treatment of malignant hypertension with 100 mg of atenolol by mouth. Reproduced with permission from Bannan LT, Beevers DG. Emergency treatment of high blood pressure with oral atenolol. *BMJ* 1981;**282**:1757–8.

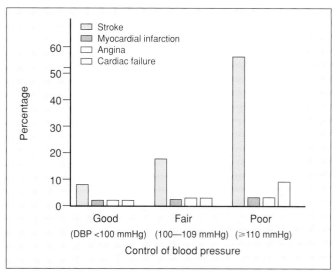

Figure 10.6 Frequency of vascular events in treated hypertensive patients following a stroke. Data from Beevers DG, Fairman MJ, Hamilton M, Harpur JE. Antihypertensive treatment in the course of established cerebrovascular disease. *Lancet* 1973;**i**:1407–8.

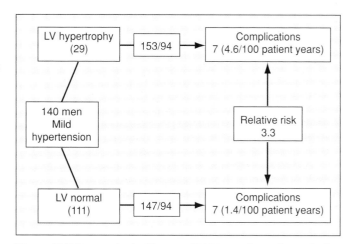

Figure 10.7 Prognostic significance of LVH on echocardiography in hypertensive patients. Reproduced from Casale PN, Devereux RB, Milner M *et al.* Value of echocardiographic measurements of left ventricular mass in predicting cardiovascular morbid events in hypertensive men. *Ann Intern Med* 1986;**105**:173–8.

promoting effect on cardiac muscle mediated by tissue renin-angiotensin systems. Furthermore, aldosterone may accelerate cardiac fibrosis. Prospective studies are needed to demonstrate whether the reduction in LVH that leads to a reduction in cardiovascular mortality and morbidity independently of any reduction in blood pressure.

Ischaemic heart disease

Both angina and myocardial infarction are common in patients with hypertension. Anginal chest pain may result from coronary artery atheroma, although at times it can result from relative ischaemia when severe LVH is not accompanied by a parallel increase in the coronary blood supply. Many patients with angina and hypertension have normal coronary arteries on angiography. Effective management of hypertension may improve a patient's anginal symptoms regardless of the drugs used. However, the drugs of choice are those with antianginal properties: the beta-blockers and the dihydropyridine calcium channel blockers, which can be used in combination if necessary. The combination of a beta-blocker with verapamil is contraindicated, because it can result in asystole, heart block, or cardiac failure. Some caution is also required when using diltiazem with a beta-blocker.

Immediately following a myocardial infarction, all patients should receive aspirin and a beta-blocker, unless these drugs are contraindicated, because these have been shown in many studies to reduce the reinfarction rate. In patients following myocardial infarction with preserved systolic function and where beta-blockers are contraindicated, there may be some benefit in using verapamil as an alternative. Similarly, diltiazem may be beneficial following non-Q wave infarctions. Dihydropyridines (particularly nifedipine) should be avoided in the immediate postinfarction state and in unstable angina.

There is increasing evidence that the ACE inhibitors are of value in patients following a myocardial infarction, particularly if there is evidence of compromised left ventricular function. In addition, reinfarction rates may be reduced. Great care is necessary, however, to avoid excessive falls in blood pressure, particularly if diuretic therapy is being prescribed concomitantly.

It is important to remember that there is a higher incidence of silent ischaemia or myocardial infarction in hypertensive patients and that in the acute stages of myocardial infarction, blood pressure may have fallen so that the diagnosis of hypertension may be missed and only become apparent at subsequent clinic visits. In addition, hypertensive patients on thiazide diuretics admitted with myocardial infarction should have their potassium concentrations checked because they may have hypokalaemia, which can exacerbate the tendency to arrhythmias and sudden death.

Heart failure

Hypertensive patients may develop heart failure as a result of either coronary heart disease or, occasionally, severe hypertension alone. Obviously, other forms of heart disease can occur and, in hypertensive patients, alcohol excess could provide a common aetiology. Echocardiography is mandatory in order to aid in the diagnosis of structural heart disease and to assess cardiac function.

The use of verapamil for hypertension in patients with heart failure is contraindicated and caution should be used with diltiazem. The accepted treatment for heart failure with

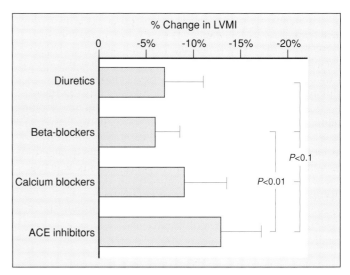

Figure 10.8 LVH regression: meta-analysis confined to double blind randomised controlled clinical studies with parallel group analysis. LVMI = Left ventricular mass index. Reproduced with permission from Schmieder RE, Martus P, Klingbeil A. Reversal of left ventricular hypertrophy in essential hypertension. A meta-analysis of randomized double-blind studies. *JAMA* 1996;**275**:1507–13.

Hypertensive patients after myocardial infarction

1. If blood pressure falls—outcome poor
2. Other risk factors often present—smoking, hyperlipidaemia, diabetes, etc.—which should be addressed
3. Consider drugs with secondary prevention properties, to reduce the rate of reinfarction:
   - Aspirin
   - Beta-blockers
   - Verapamil or diltiazem—limited data, as second line agents if beta-blockers contraindicated and good left ventricular function
   - ACE inhibitors—especially for patients with LV impairment
   - Statins—if serum cholesterol >5.0 mmol
4. Care with some drugs needed because of
   - Low blood pressure
   - Heart failure

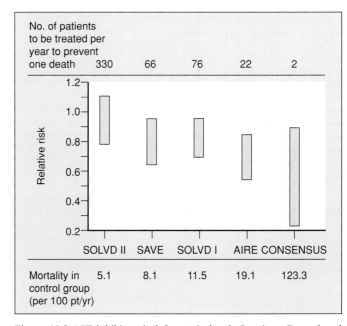

Figure 10.9 ACE inhibitors in left ventricular dysfunction. Reproduced with permission from Davey-Smith G, Egger M. *BMJ* 1994;**308**:72–4.

diuretics and ACE inhibitors could well bring the patient's blood pressure under control. The ACE inhibitors have been proven in many trials to prolong life in patients with heart failure, so they are probably the drugs of first choice for patients with heart failure and hypertension. A similar although smaller benefit is also seen using a combination of hydralazine and nitrates; however, this combination is not commonly used unless ACE inhibitors are contraindicated or cause side effects. Recent evidence has also suggested that careful use of beta-blockers, such as carvedilol, bisoprolol and metoprolol, may improve the prognosis in patients with heart failure secondary to systolic impairment, especially by reducing the risk of arrhythmias and sudden cardiac death. Another recent randomised controlled trial (RALES) has demonstrated that the aldosterone antagonist, spironolactone, also significantly reduced mortality and morbidity.

Peripheral vascular disease

A strong association exists between peripheral vascular disease and hypertension, which is exacerbated by increases in serum lipid concentrations and by smoking. Although control of blood pressure is important in these patients, caution needs to be exercised with some drugs, particularly the beta-blockers, which may worsen symptoms in patients with rest pain. Randomised trials have shown that the careful use of cardioselective beta-blockers does not significantly alter claudication distance.

In addition, the presence of peripheral vascular disease may increase the likelihood of an undiagnosed atheromatous renal artery stenosis, with the consequence that the use of ACE inhibitors needs careful monitoring. In patients with peripheral vascular disease, an "exquisite" or over rapid fall in blood pressure in response to ACE inhibitor, or a significant rise in serum creatinine levels, raises a strong possibility of underlying renal artery stenosis. Renal angiography should seriously be considered. Calcium channel blockers are probably the drugs of first choice because they are relatively safe in peripheral vascular disease and, in fact, they may modestly improve the symptoms of claudication.

Renal disease

Hypertensive patients with elevated serum creatinine levels or proteinuria may have parenchymal or obstructive renal disease, and should be referred for specialist evaluation. Renovascular disease (renal artery stenosis) is relatively uncommon, but may be the most frequent curable cause of hypertension. In patients with chronic renal impairment, hypertension also accelerates the rate of loss of renal function, and good blood pressure control is essential to retard this process. Routine investigation of all hypertensive patients is not justifiable, but doctors should be aware of important clues suggesting renal disease.

Malignant hypertension can cause rapid loss of renal function that can be irreversible if untreated. Otherwise there is some debate whether essential hypertension alone can cause

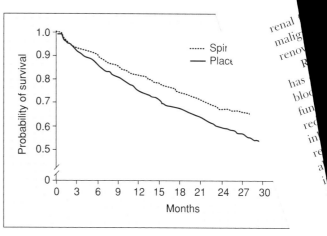

Figure 10.10 Survival curve for randomised aldactone evaluation study (RALES) showing 30% reduction in all cause mortality when spironolactone (up to 25 mg) was added to conventional treatment in patients with severe (New York Heart Association class IV) chronic heart failure. Reproduced from Pitt B, Zanad F, Remmie WJ *et al.* The effects of spironolactone or morbidity and mortality in patients with severe heart failure. *N Engl J Med* 1999;**341**:709–17.

Antihypertensive drugs and peripheral vascular disease

- Beta-blockers may worsen claudication
- ACE inhibitors hazardous if renal artery stenosis present
- Thiazides raise lipids and glucose (small effect)
- Calcium channel blockers may relieve symptoms
- Lipid lowering drugs often necessary
- Type 2 diabetes mellitus often present

Patients with peripheral vascular disease may have undiagnosed renal artery stenosis

---

Table 10.1 Renal artery stenosis: Mayo Clinic. Reproduced with permission from Hunt JC, Strong CG. Renovascular hypertension. Mechanisms, natural history and treatment. *Am J Cardiol* 1973;**32**:562–74.

	Atheroma	Fibromuscular dysplasia
Age (yr)	53 (35–73)	39 (6–64)
M:F	65:35	27–73
Proportion (%)	65	35
Bruit (%)	40	80
Bilateral (%)	31	24
CHD/CVA (%)	49	Rare
Developed renal failure (%)	15	Rare
5-year survival (%)	67	92
Disease progression (%)	28	—

Primary renal diseases causing hypertension

- IgA nephropathy
- Pyelonephritis
- Membranous retinopathy
- Mesangioproliferative glomerulonephritis
- Adult polycystic kidney disease
- Vasculitis
- Henoch–Schölein purpura

...failure, and thus renal impairment in the absence of ...nant hypertension suggests primary renal disease or ...ascular disease.

...egardless of the cause of renal impairment, hypertension ...considerable influence over its progression, with good ...od pressure control slowing the deterioration in renal ...ction. Meta-analysis of all controlled trials showed a 30% ...uction in incidence of end-stage renal failure with ACE ...hibitors. Whether ACE inhibitors have a specific ...noprotective effect in non-diabetic renal failure, over and ...bove their antihypertensive action, remains uncertain. ACE ...hibitors reduce microproteinuria and macroproteinuria, and ...re renoprotective in patients with proteinuria >3 g/day due to various forms of glomerulonephritis or nephropathy but not in polycystic kidney disease. ACE inhibitors may cause or worsen renal impairment in patients with critical renovascular disease, so they should be used with caution in patients with advanced chronic renal impairment. Blood pressure is particularly salt sensitive in patients with impaired renal function, and dietary salt reduction is important.

Calcium channel blockers are effective and relatively safe for treating hypertension in patients with renal failure. Thiazide diuretics may be ineffective in patients with mild renal impairment, and loop diuretics (frusemide), often in high dose, are frequently required. Caution is needed in patients with renal failure who are receiving diuretic therapy because, if they become dehydrated, the ACE inhibitors may precipitate large falls in blood pressure. Any drugs that are excreted by the kidney (in particular, ACE inhibitors and some beta-blockers) need to be given initially in reduced doses.

Based on the 1999 British Hypertension Society guidelines, the threshold for antihypertensive treatment in patients with renal disease is >140 mmHg systolic, or >90 mmHg diastolic for patients with persistent proteinuria or renal impairment. Optimal blood pressure control is <130/85 mmHg, and reducing blood pressure to <125/75 mmHg may produce additional benefit in patients with chronic renal disease of any aetiology and proteinuria of >1 g/24 hours. Patients with renal failure have a very high risk of cardiovascular complications, and may need aspirin or statin treatment in addition to non-pharmacological measures to reduce their exaggerated cardiovascular risk burden.

Patients with end-stage renal failure, and those on dialysis or following transplantation, also have a particularly high incidence of atheromatous vascular disease, heart attacks, and strokes. Hypertension is also almost universal, but usually easily controlled with dialysis. In patients who are anuric, salt and water restriction between dialyses may maintain blood pressure control, although in some patients drug therapy is still needed. Patients with end-stage renal failure are usually anaemic, and this can be corrected by treatment with erythropoietin. However, this treatment is associated with a rise in blood pressure, perhaps related to increases in renin, haematocrit and blood volume.

Renal transplantation may obviate the need for dialysis, but a high proportion of transplant recipients develop hypertension. This is more common in patients who have received kidneys from hypertensive donors. Post-transplant hypertension in the early phase may be related to acute rejection or acute tubular necrosis, which follows the ischaemic period. There may be a component of fluid overload if the patient was underdialysed before the operation, and the use of corticosteroids as immunosuppressive agents can exacerbate this. In the long term, the use of cyclosporin A may also cause hypertension, possibly due to enhancement of the effects of renin and angiotensin II.

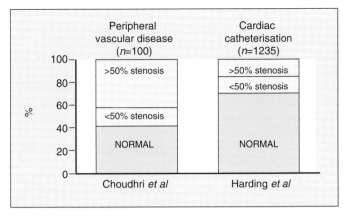

Figure 10.11 The frequency of previously undiagnosed renal artery stenosis in patients with peripheral vascular disease (Choudhri AH, Cleland JG, Rowlands PC et al. Unsuspected renal artery stenosis in peripheral vascular disease. *BMJ* 1990;**301**:1197–8.) or undergoing cardiac catheterisation (Harding MB, Smith LR, Himmelstein SI et al. Renal artery stenosis: prevalence and associated risk factors in patients undergoing routine cardiac catheterization. *J Am Soc Nephrol* 1992;**2**:1608–16).

Clues suggesting renovascular disease

- Onset of hypertension before the age of 30
- Young females (fibromuscular dysplasia)
- Documented sudden onset of hypertension or recent worsening of hypertension in middle age
- Accelerated (malignant) hypertension
- Resistant hypertension (to a three drug regimen)
- Renal impairment of unknown cause
- Excessive fall in blood pressure or elevation of serum creatinine by ACE inhibitor or angiotensin II antagonist treatment
- Peripheral vascular disease or severe generalised atherosclerotic disease
- Recurrent pulmonary oedema or heart failure with no obvious cause

Patients with any of these features should be referred for specialist advice because the investigations required to confirm or exclude renovascular disease are complex.

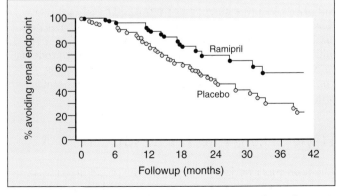

Figure 10.12 Ramipril vs placebo in non-diabetic nephropathy. Reproduced with permission from *Lancet* 1997;**349**:1857

Hypertension can develop in response to renin secretion from the patient's own atrophic kidneys, or exaggerated atheromatous renal artery stenosis may affect the transplanted kidney; occasionally, stenosis can also occur at the surgical anastomosis. Whatever happens, adequate blood pressure control is required to preserve functioning of the transplanted kidney.

Hyperlipidaemia

Hyperlipidaemia when present in combination with hypertension confers a greatly increased cardiovascular risk. Fifty per cent of hypertensive patients also have hyperlipidaemia, and the risk is particularly increased with higher plasma cholesterol concentrations and low density lipoprotein concentrations. Treatment of this hyperlipidaemia should be with stringent dietetic advice, which can bring about an average 5% reduction in serum total cholesterol. Very often lipid lowering drugs have to be used in addition. Antihypertensive drugs should be selected based on their effects on serum lipids. Thiazides and beta-blockers may have adverse effects on lipid profiles, whereas alpha-blockers may be beneficial. Calcium channel blockers and ACE inhibitors are lipid neutral.

In our view, hypertensive patients who have hyperlipidaemia must be considered at particularly high risk of heart attack or stroke, so an active lipid lowering strategy is necessary. In several controlled outcome trials, statin treatment for secondary and primary prevention reduced major coronary events by 30%, as well as all cause mortality significantly, and is safe, simple, and well tolerated. In the trials, statin therapy also reduces the risk of stroke by about a third. In sub-group analyses of the large trials, the benefits were similar in hypertensive patients. There is general acceptance that statin treatment should be targeted at a specified threshold of coronary risk, and not at thresholds of lipid values. The main constraints on statin treatment at present are the workload for general practitioners and the enormous potential cost. Use of lipid lowering therapy in hypertensive patients is discussed further in Chapter 9.

Connective tissue diseases

Rheumatoid arthritis, systemic lupus erythematosus, polyarteritis nodosa, and the other connective tissue disorders are all associated with renal damage and hypertension, which may be worsened through the use of non-steroidal anti-inflammatory drugs, corticosteroids, and gold therapy. These treatments can raise blood pressure even further or interfere with the action of antihypertensive drugs. Overall, the most suitable drugs seem to be calcium channel blockers and ACE inhibitors, with some studies suggesting that the ACE inhibitors may protect the kidney in patients with scleroderma. In these patients careful monitoring of renal function is important, and renal involvement should be suspected if proteinuria is detected.

Hypertension and anaesthesia

The problems associated with hypertension and anaesthesia can be divided into those relating to the evaluation of the blood pressure itself and those relating to the use of antihypertensive agents. Important factors to also consider are

Drugs in renal disease	
ACE inhibitors	Care when used in conjunction with diuretic therapy for renal failure
	Small doses initially
	Probably renoprotective in the long term
Beta-blockers	Small doses initially
Calcium channel blockers	Relatively safe in patients with renal failure
Loop diuretics	Useful in cases of sodium or water retention

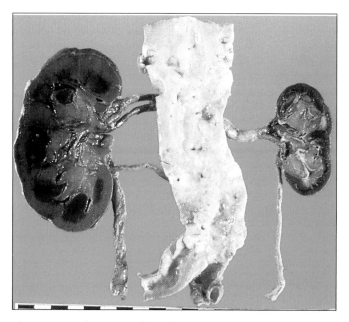

Figure 10.13 The aorta and renal arteries from a patient with severe hypertension and hyperlipidaemia

The most suitable drugs for patients with connective tissue diseases
• Calcium channel blockers
• ACE inhibitors
• Alpha-blockers

whether or not hypotensive anaesthesia is planned, and whether major or minor surgery is contemplated.

Patients who have mild symptomless hypertension, and who are otherwise fit, are at no particular risk in the perioperative period. Many non-urgent surgical operations are postponed unnecessarily. In particular, many patients may be considered to be hypertensive when, in fact, they are exhibiting "white coat" hypertension associated with anxiety caused by admission to hospital. By contrast, patients who have sustained severe hypertension are at risk of perioperative arrhythmias or myocardial infarctions. In these patients elective surgery should be postponed if blood pressure >180/110 and/or LVH is present on the ECG, until they have been fully assessed and their blood pressure controlled.

Anaesthesia and surgery can exacerbate problems in those patients taking particular antihypertensive medication; for example, the beta-blockers may block the compensatory rise in heart rate associated with fluid loss and the ACE inhibitors may block the response of the renin-angiotensin system, with the result that patients taking these drugs are prone to hypotension following blood loss. However, beta-blockers should not be stopped in the perioperative period, particularly in patients with coronary artery disease, because this may provoke myocardial ischaemia. The important point in the management of these patients is for the anaesthetist to be aware that the patient is taking these drugs.

In those cases where antihypertensive drugs have to be stopped because the patient should not take them, they should be started again as soon as possible. Parenteral control of hypertension is, however, seldom indicated because patients are usually resting in bed and receiving opioid analgesia which may, in fact, reduce blood pressure.

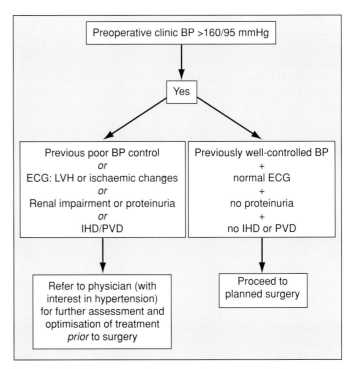

Figure 10.14 Management of preoperative hypertension in a patient undergoing elective surgery

Hypertension in children

Hypertension is an uncommon problem in children and, where present, it is almost invariably the result of underlying causes. In particular, there may be renal or arteritic diseases. There is a need for more information on hypertension in children, and much of the present knowledge is based on paediatric nephrology and a small number of epidemiological studies.

Blood pressures rise sharply as children mature and those children who have higher blood pressures to start with tend to show a faster rise with advancing age. This is a particular problem in obese children. It is probable that the origins of adult essential hypertension are to be found in childhood or even infancy.

At the present state of knowledge, it is not considered justifiable to attempt to screen the blood pressure in all children. However, children who have any evidence of systemic illness should have their blood pressure measured. Under the age of three years, blood pressure measurement can only be achieved with Doppler flow equipment and, of course, at all ages, the appropriate size cuff must be employed. The Second Task Force on Blood Pressure Control in Children suggests that all physicians who care for children 3 years of age through adolescence should be encouraged to measure blood pressures once a year. Current guidelines suggest that blood pressure should be measured with the child in a comfortable sitting position (although infants may be supine), with the right arm exposed and supported at the heart level. However, phase V sounds may be difficult to obtain in children, and the Second Task Force guidelines discuss K4 diastolic blood pressures in the standards for infants and children 3–12 years

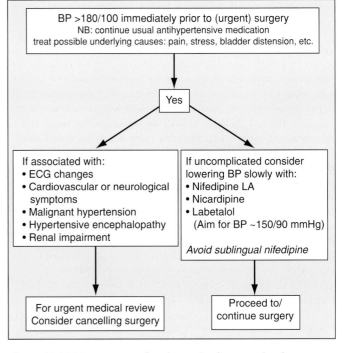

Figure 10.15 Management of perioperative hypertension in a patient undergoing urgent surgery

of age, and K5 diastolic blood pressures for adolescents 13–18 years of age. More recently the update on the Second Task Force favours phase K5 diastolic pressure at all ages. We suggest that the position of the subject during measurement, the limb and cuff size used should all be recorded, as well as the fourth and fifth Korotkoff diastolic sounds if both are heard.

Children whose blood pressures exceed the 90th percentile for their age need careful rechecking, and if they exceed the 95th percentile they need referral to hospital specialists and a detailed investigation. However apart from non-pharmacological therapy, particularly with salt restriction and correction/avoidance of obesity, the beta-blockers, calcium antagonists, and alpha-blockers are generally safe. The thiazides however have long term metabolic effects and should generally be avoided as prolonged monotherapy in children. In addition, the ACE inhibitors should also be used with caution in children with renal disease. Nevertheless, in the present survey, a significant number of paediatricians would prescribe thiazides and the ACE inhibitors as first line therapy.

Hypertension in older patients

The topic of hypertension in the elderly has undergone a major change over the last 15 years. There is now abundant evidence that this group in particular benefit more from antihypertensive therapy than younger patients. Apart from this, hypertension in the elderly does not differ from hypertension in general. The assessment of a hypertensive patient at any age should not differ and the concept of "the elderly" being a special group should be abandoned.

Systolic blood pressure rises steadily with increasing age, and the prevalence of hypertension including isolated systolic hypertension (that is, systolic blood pressure >160 and diastolic blood pressure <90 mmHg) is more than 50% in those over 60 years. These people have a high risk of cardiovascular complications when compared to younger hypertensives, and antihypertensive treatment of isolated systolic and systolic-diastolic hypertension reduces this risk.

Antihypertensive therapy in the elderly also reduces the incidence of heart failure by 50% and also reduces dementia, which are important complications of hypertension in this age group. Before these outcome trials it was a widely and incorrectly held view that a rise in blood pressure with age was inevitable and harmless, and that isolated systolic hypertension was of no consequence. Evidence for benefit from antihypertensive treatment extends until at least the age of 80 years, and regular blood pressure screening should continue until this age. When hypertension is first diagnosed beyond the age of 80 there is no firm evidence to guide policy, but decisions should probably be based on biological rather than chronological age, especially in patients who are generally fit and have a reasonable life expectancy, particularly if they have hypertensive complications or target organ damage.

Meta-analysis of the subgroups of patients over the age of 80 years suggests that antihypertensive treatment is effective particularly at preventing strokes. An ongoing trial (HYVET) comparing an ACE inhibitor based regime with placebo is currently underway. In the meantime it seems wise to prescribe antihypertensive drugs if the blood pressure exceeds 180/100 mmHg or there is evidence of end-organ damage (LVH, angina, post infarction, previous stroke). However while there remains some uncertainty on the value of drug treatment, it is indefensible to cause drug side effects. The thiazide diuretics remain the drugs of first choice as they have very few side effects.

Table 10.2 Definition of high blood pressure in children. Data taken from Report of the Second Task Force on Blood Pressure Control in Children. *Pediatrics* 1987;**79**:1–25.

Term	Definition
Normal blood pressure	Systolic and diastolic blood pressures <90th percentile for age and sex
High normal blood pressure	Average systolic and/or diastolic blood pressure between 90th and 95th percentiles for age and sex
High blood pressure (hypertension)	Average systolic and/or diastolic blood pressures <95th percentile for age and sex with measurements obtained on at least three occasions

All children with blood pressure >140/90 should be referred to a paediatrician with an interest in hypertension

Table 10.3 Classification of hypertension by age group. Data taken from Report of the Second Task Force on Blood Pressure Control in Children. *Pediatrics* 1987;**79**:1–25.

Age group	Significant hypertension (mmHg)	Severe hypertension (mmHg)
Newborn	Systolic BP ≥ 96	Systolic BP ≥ 106
8–30 days	Systolic BP ≥ 104	Systolic BP ≥ 110
Infant (<2 yr)	Systolic BP ≥ 112	Systolic BP ≥ 118
	Diastolic BP ≥ 74	Diastolic BP ≥ 82
Children (3–5 yr)	Systolic BP ≥ 116	Systolic BP ≥ 124
	Diastolic BP ≥ 76	Diastolic BP ≥ 84
Children (6–9 yr)	Systolic BP ≥ 122	Systolic BP ≥ 130
	Diastolic BP ≥ 78	Diastolic BP ≥ 86
Children (10–12 yr)	Systolic BP ≥ 126	Systolic BP ≥ 134
	Diastolic BP ≥ 82	Diastolic BP ≥ 90
Adolescents (13–15 yr)	Systolic BP ≥ 136	Systolic BP ≥ 144
	Diastolic BP ≥ 86	Diastolic BP ≥ 92
Adolescents (16–18 yr)	Systolic BP ≥ 142	Systolic BP ≥ 150
	Diastolic BP ≥ 92	Diastolic BP ≥ 98

Hypertension in older patients

- Older hypertensive patients should not be treated differently from younger ones; they are not a separate "sub group"
- Antihypertensive treatment has been validated up to the age of 80 years. The thresholds for starting treatment and the targets for BP reduction are the same for all ages
- Above the age of 80 there is strong evidence that treatment is worthwhile although no dedicated trial in such patients is available yet
- There is a tendency for the thiazide diuretics and the calcium blockers to be the most effective first-line therapy

Table 10.4 Reduction in mortality and morbidity of older patients.

| | Percentage of cases prevented† (95% confidence interval) | | | |
	Cardiovascular events*	Stroke	Coronary heart disease	All cause mortality
Mortality	30% (19–39)	40% (21–54)	26% (14–36)	16% (6–25)
Morbidity	NC	35% (24–45)	15% (1–27)	NA
Combined M/M	33% (25–41)	37% (28–45)	20% (10–30)	NA

*Cardiovascular = both strokes and CHD events including sudden death

†Treated for approximately 5 years, reduction compared to controls. Patients were largely ambulatory outpatients, although not exclusively, and treated for 2–7 years. Mean blood pressure at study entry across all studies was 177/90 mmHg (includes patients with isolated systolic hypertension in some studies)

The mean reduction blood pressure at the end of study was 13.3 mmHg systolic and 7.7 mmHg diastolic

NA = not applicable, NC = not calculated

Elderly hypertensives respond to non-pharmacological measures to lower blood pressure at least as well as younger patients. Antihypertensive therapy is indicated and clearly beneficial in people aged 60 years or more, when blood pressure averages are >160 mmHg systolic and >90 mmHg diastolic. For systolic blood pressures 140–159 mmHg and diastolic blood pressures <90 mmHg (borderline isolated systolic hypertension), treatment is advised when there are cardiovascular complications or evidence of target organ damage. The treatment of choice in elderly hypertensives is a low dose thiazide diuretic. Beta-blockers were second line agents in many of the outcome trials, but are less effective than thiazides in the elderly. Indeed, the beta-blockers decrease stroke but no other cardiovascular events in this age group. In the SYST-Eur (Systolic Hypertension-Europe) trial, treatment of isolated systolic hypertension in elderly patients used the dihydropyridine calcium antagonist, nitrendipine, and the outcome was similar to that with diuretic based treatment in SHEP (Systolic Hypertension in the Elderly Program).

Oral contraceptives and hypertension

The combined oral contraceptives pills (OCP) have a small adverse effect on blood pressure with average increases of 5/3 mmHg. In a small proportion of women (~1%) severe hypertension may be induced, including cases of malignant hypertension. The increase in blood pressure appears to be idiosyncratic in that it may occur many months or years after first using a combined OCP. No particular sub-groups of OCP users have been clearly identified as being susceptible to blood pressure increases and the cause for the blood pressure has not been established. Moreover, the dose related effects of oestrogens and progestogens on blood pressure have not been clearly established. As the blood pressure response to any combined OCP preparation is unpredictable, and there is a small increase in cardiovascular risk associated with OCP use, blood pressure should always be measured before starting OCP use and then six monthly thereafter.

The oral progestogen-only contraceptive pills (POPs) do not usually induce an increase in blood pressure. The POPs have therefore been recommended for use in women with a previous history of combined OCP-induced hypertension, or those women with hypertension wishing to use an oral contraceptive.

The combined OCP is not absolutely contraindicated for women who are already hypertensive or those who develop hypertension during use of combined OCPs. However, other non-hormonal forms of contraception should be considered, especially if other risk factors for cardiovascular disease (e.g., smoking or migraine) coexist. In those women for whom other methods of contraception are unacceptable, changing to a

Table 10.5 Reduction in morbidity of patients aged 80+ years. Data taken from Gueyffier F, Bulpitt C, Boissel JP *et al*. Antihypertensive drugs in very old people: a subgroup meta-analysis of randomized controlled trials. INDANA Group. *Lancet* 1999;**353**:793–6.

| | Percentage of cases prevented* (95% confidence interval) | | |
	Cardiovascular events†	Stroke	Heart failure
Morbidity	22% (2–60)	34% (10–52)	39% (10–60)

*Treated for approximately 3.5 years, reduction compared to controls. Patients were largely ambulatory outpatients, although not exclusively. Mean blood pressure at study entry across all studies was 180/84 mmHg (includes patients with isolated systolic hypertension in some studies). Age ranged from 80–99 years. 95% confidence intervals estimated from graph

†Cardiovascular = both strokes and CHD events

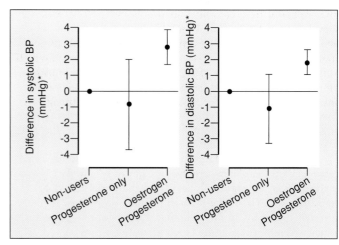

Figure 10.16 Blood pressure and oral contraceptives. *Adjusted for confounding variables. Reproduced from Dong W, Colhoun HM, Paulter NR. Blood pressure in women using oral contraceptives: results from the Health Survey for England 1994. *J Hypertens* 1997;**15**:1063–8.

POP with careful monitoring of blood pressure is recommended. If blood pressure does not fall below 160/100 mmHg, antihypertensive medication should be initiated. Many women are wrongly told that they cannot be given an OCP on the basis of mild transient or sustained elevations of blood pressure. The hazards of an unwanted pregnancy far outweigh the tiny increase in cardiovascular risk induced by the OCP.

Hormone replacement therapy and hypertension

Most studies on the effects of hormone replacement therapy (HRT) on blood pressure have been conducted in normotensive women. In such patients, two studies have observed a significant reduction in diastolic blood pressure during treatment with combined oestrogen and progesterone HRT, whereas systolic blood pressure remained unchanged. We are only aware of three studies investigating the effects of HRT in hypertensive women. The retrospective study by Pfeffer *et al.* included 35 women (aged 52–87) with documented hypertension, in whom a fall in systolic blood pressure was demonstrated with oral oestrogen therapy. In a small prospective Danish study, 12 normotensive and 12 hypertensive women were started on HRT and followed up for one year, and a fall in systolic blood pressure was demonstrated in the hypertensive group. Our large open prospective study demonstrated that HRT did not adversely affect blood pressure in 75 hypertensive women despite an average gain in weight. These data strongly suggest that menopausal women with hypertension need not be denied the benefits of HRT for the amelioration of vasomotor symptoms and also the possible benefits against cardiovascular disease and osteoporosis.

The average British general practitioner has about 50 female patients on his list aged 40–59 years, of whom five might be expected to be hypertensive. In view of the lack of consensus in the prescribing habits of HRT, we would suggest the following guidelines. All clinicians should measure blood pressure before starting HRT. In a normotensive postmenopausal woman, blood pressure should be measured annually following the start of HRT. One exception may be the use of Premarin in high dose, where a follow up blood pressure measurement should be made at three months, in view of reports of a possible rare idiosyncratic rise in blood pressure. In hypertensive menopausal women, blood pressure should at least be measured initially and thereafter six monthly, although if blood pressure is labile or difficult to control, three monthly measurements should be carried out. If a hypertensive woman on HRT demonstrates a rise in blood pressure, careful monitoring or observation and perhaps an alteration or increase of their antihypertensive treatment should be given.

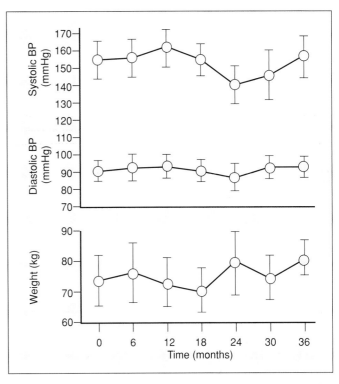

Figure 10.17 Sequential changes in blood pressure and weight in 75 hypertensive women taking hormone replacement therapy. Reproduced with permission from Lip GYH, Beevers M, Churchill D, Beevers DG. Hormone replacement therapy and blood pressure in hypertensive women. *J Hum Hypertens* 1994;**8**:491–4.

Further reading

- Edmunds E, Lip GYH. Cardiovascular risk in women: the cardiologists perspective. *Q J Med* 2000;**93**:135–45.
- Gibbs C, Beevers DG, Lip GYH. The management of hypertensive disease in black patients. *Q J Med* 1999;**92**:187–92.
- The Sixth Report of the Joint National Committee on prevention, detection, evaluation and treatment of high blood pressure (JNC-V1). *Arch Intern Med* 1997;**157**:2413–46.
- Update on the 1987 Task Force on High Blood Pressure in Children and Adolescents. *Pediatrics* 1996;**98**:647–58.

11 Diabetes and hypertension

Hypertension and diabetes mellitus commonly occur together, and as they are both associated with hyperlipidaemia; this means that many patients will have three cardiovascular risk factors even if they do not smoke. All these factors should be addressed aggressively because their synergistic effects put the patient at greater cardiovascular risk.

> Major changes in our understanding of the importance of high blood pressure in diabetic patients have occurred since 1995

Epidemiology

The prevalence of hypertension differs in type 1 and type 2 diabetes. In type 1 diabetes, in the absence of nephropathy (microalbuminuria or proteinuria), the prevalence of hypertension is similar to that in the non-diabetic population. In type 2 diabetes, hypertension (>140/90 mmHg) is present in over 70% of patients. The aetiology of hypertension in diabetes is much debated.

Pathophysiology

In insulin dependent diabetes (IDDM), it is believed to result mainly from diabetic renal disease with activation of the renin-angiotensin system. In non-insulin dependent diabetes (NIDDM), the situation is less clear, although there seems to be volume expansion with sodium retention, which may be related to hyperinsulinaemia, and the patients are often obese.

Patients with diabetes suffer from both macrovascular complications, such as myocardial infarction and peripheral vascular disease, and microvascular disease, such as diabetic nephropathy and retinopathy. Hypertension aggravates both macro- and microvascular complications of diabetes. Thus the presence of diabetes in hypertensives not only substantially adds to their cardiovascular and stroke risk, which is more than would be expected from either risk factor alone, but has implications for choice of therapy. Proteinuria on Dipstix testing is associated with a poor prognosis; this also appears to be the case for microproteinuria (urine albumin between 20 and 200 mg/24 hours), which can be detected before Dipstix testing becomes positive.

Both diabetes and hypertension are commonly associated with cardiovascular complications such as heart failure and atrial fibrillation, although the underlying vascular disease may be the common denominator. In atrial fibrillation, both diabetes and/or hypertension substantially increase the risk of stroke and thromboembolism. There remains some debate as to whether there is a separate clinical syndrome of diabetic cardiomyopathy.

Management

Perhaps the most important recent lesson in the treatment of diabetic hypertensives is that tighter blood pressure control saves lives. Both the HOT (Hypertension Optimal Treatment) study and UKPDS (United Kingdom Prospective Diabetes Study) found significantly lower rates of adverse events in those achieving the lowest target blood pressures. Accordingly, the target blood pressure in patients with diabetes should now be 130/85 mmHg or lower.

Table 11.1 Risk factors for CHD in non-insulin dependent diabetes mellitus (NIDDM) in the UKPDS. Data reproduced from Turner RC, Millns H, Neil HA *et al. BMJ* 1998;**316**:823–8.

Rank	CHD (280)	Myocardial infarction: fatal + non-fatal (192)	Fatal myocardial infarction (79)
First	LDL-C	LDL-C	DBP
Second	HDL-C	DBP	LDL-C
Third	HbA$_{1C}$	Smoking	HbA$_{1c}$
Fourth	SBP	HDL-C	
Fifth	Smoking	HbA$_{1c}$	

Baseline population: 2693 white M+F free of heart disease at entry
LDL-C = low density lipoprotein cholesterol; HbA$_{1C}$ = glycated haemoglobin; HDL-C = high density lipoprotein cholesterol

Table 11.2 Predictors of cardiovascular mortality in insulin dependent diabetes mellitus. Data reproduced from Rossing P, Hougaard P, Borch-Johnsen, K, Parving HH. Predictors of mortality in insulin dependent diabetes: 10 year observational follow up study. *BMJ* 1996;**313**:779–84.

Predictor of mortality	Relative risk	P
Age	1.11	<0.0001
Smoking	2.23	<0.01
Microalbuminuria	1.87	<0.05
Overt nephropathy	2.97	<0.001
Hypertension	2.25	<0.01
Glycaemic control	NS*	NS*

*NS = not significant

In general, the treatment of hypertension in diabetic patients should take into account the effects of antihypertensive drugs on glucose and lipid metabolism. Alpha-blockers are safe in diabetics and may even have a small beneficial effect on plasma lipids. Calcium channel blockers and ACE inhibitors are neutral in their effects and are also safe when used carefully. Thiazide diuretics may very slightly worsen insulin resistance and should be used with caution in non-insulin dependent diabetic patients, although, they can be used in insulin dependent diabetic patients when their effects on glucose tolerance can easily be offset by a small increase in insulin dosage. The beta-blockers are generally safe but may produce a lack of awareness of hypoglycaemic symptoms and should be used with caution. However, atenolol seems to be generally well accepted (see later).

Type 1 diabetes

These patients usually get microvascular complications (e.g., retinopathy, nephropathy) rather than macrovascular disease, and importantly they are insulin deficient and usually young. Hypertension in type 1 diabetes often indicates the presence of diabetic nephropathy. Blood pressure reduction and ACE inhibitor treatment slow the rate of decline of renal function in overt diabetic nephropathy and delay progression from the microalbuminuric phase to overt nephropathy. Type 1 diabetic subjects with evidence of nephropathy are at very high risk of cardiovascular disease and may be considered for statin therapy if their total cholesterol is >5 mmol/L and aspirin therapy if they satisfy the criteria set out by the BHS.

The threshold for intervention with antihypertensive therapy in diabetic patients without evidence of nephropathy is a systolic blood pressure of <140/90 mmHg, and the optimal blood pressure target is <140/80 mmHg. The target blood pressure is <130/80 mmHg (or lower <125/75 mmHg) when there is evidence of proteinuria >1 g/24 hours.

In type 1 diabetes, there is evidence that ACE inhibitors reduce the progression of nephropathy and possibly even retinopathy and neuropathy. These drugs should thus be regarded as first line agents in hypertensive diabetic patients with these complications. It is possible that type 1 diabetic subjects with persistent microalbuminuria or proteinuria and "normal" blood pressures may also benefit from ACE inhibition titrated to the recommended maximum dose. If ACE inhibitor treatment has to be discontinued because of persistent cough, an angiotensin II receptor antagonist may be considered, although evidence for specific renoprotection by this drug class is awaited from ongoing clinical trials. For renoprotection blood pressure control is most important, and combinations of antihypertensive drugs are invariably required to achieve recommended blood pressure targets.

Type 2 diabetes

These patients are usually older than patients with type 1 diabetes, and are insulin resistant and prone to macrovascular complications, such as coronary artery disease, stroke, and peripheral vascular disease. Microvascular disease is less common and thus type 2 diabetes is more of a cardiovascular risk factor. In type 2 diabetes, hypertension is strongly related to but not fully accounted for by obesity, and is highly predictive of cardiovascular and microvascular complications. Hypertension accelerates the decline of renal function in type 2 diabetic patients with established nephropathy. This decline is slowed by antihypertensive therapy particularly with the ACE inhibitors.

> Analysis of the results of UKPDS and the diabetic sub-groups in HOT, SHEP and SYST-EUR suggest that diabetics obtain more benefit from antihypertensive treatment than non-diabetics

> Similarly, diabetic myocardial infarct survivors obtain more benefit from lipid lowering than non-diabetics (The 4S Study)

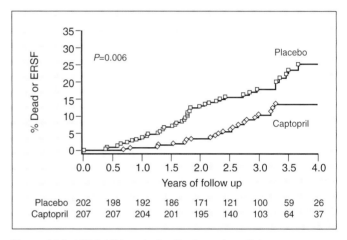

Figure 11.1 ACE inhibitors in insulin dependent diabetes. Reproduced with permission from Lewis EJ, Hunsicker LG, Bain RP, Rohde RD, for the Collaborative Study Group. The effect of angiotensin-converting-enzyme inhibition on diabetic nephropathy. *New Engl J Med* 1993;**329**:1456–62.

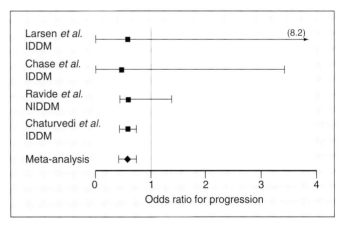

Figure 11.2 ACE inhibitors and diabetic retinopathy. Reproduced with permission from Chaturvedi N, Sjolie AK, Stephenson JM *et al.* Effect of lisinopril on progression of retinopathy in normotensive people with type I diabetes. The EUCLID Study Group. EURODIAB Controlled Trial of Lisinopril in Insulin-Dependent Diabetes Mellitus *Lancet* 1998;**351**:28–31.

Insights from the United Kingdom Prospective Diabetes Study (UKPDS)

The UKPDS examined two facets of hypertension care in diabetics: first, whether tighter blood pressure control might reduce both adverse events and the progression of end-organ damage and second, in view of reports that ACE inhibitors might be particularly beneficial in diabetic hypertensives, whether the ACE inhibitor captopril was more effective in preventing diabetic complications than the beta-blocker atenolol.

The UKPDS found that in the sub-group of diabetics who also had hypertension, tight blood pressure control, attaining a mean blood pressure of 144/82 mmHg, compared with 154/87 mmHg using either a beta-blocker or an ACE inhibitor, produced significant benefits in diabetics. There were statistically significant reductions in any diabetes related endpoint, including diabetes related death as well as reductions in the development of stroke, myocardial infarction, heart failure, microalbuminuria and progression of diabetic retinopathy in the tight blood pressure control group. Indeed, tight blood pressure control resulted in significant reductions in vascular endpoints, when compared to tight diabetic control.

Insights from the diabetic sub-group of the Hypertension Optimal Treatment (HOT) study

This large scale trial is described in detail in Chapter 2. 1501 of the participants had NIDDM, and in this sub-group those whose target blood pressure was below 80 mmHg suffered significantly less coronary heart disease at follow up compared to the patients whose targets were 85 mmHg and 90 mmHg respectively. This together with the UKPDS confirm that in hypertensive patients with diabetes aggressive blood pressure control for a target of below 140/80 mmHg is highly beneficial.

Insights from the diabetic sub-group of the SYST-Eur (Systolic Hypertension-Europe) trial

Details of this trial appear in Chapter 2. Those patients with isolated systolic hypertension also had NIDDM and those receiving treatment with a calcium channel blocker obtained numerically fewer coronary and stroke events than the non-diabetics on the same treatment. The control of systolic blood pressure in both diabetics and non-diabetics is in fact more important than the control of the diastolic blood pressure.

Choice of drugs

In type 2 diabetes, trials have demonstrated reductions in proteinuria with ACE inhibitors and calcium antagonists. However, UKPDS found no difference in reduction in either macrovascular disease such as myocardial infarction and peripheral vascular disease, or microvascular disease such as diabetic retinopathy or proteinuria, between a beta-blocker (atenolol) and an ACE inhibitor, although this trial was not powered to find a significant difference between the two regimes. Low dose diuretics have also been found to be as effective in diabetic as in non-diabetic patients. It thus appears that the benefits conferred in NIDDM by ACE inhibitors may simply be a product of blood pressure reduction, which can be attained with any antihypertensive drug.

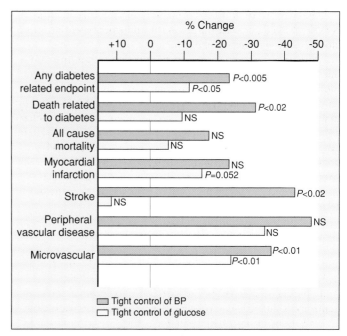

Figure 11.3 United Kingdom Prospective Diabetes Study (UKPDS) Group 1998 treatment of type 2 diabetes. Comparison of the benefits of tight blood pressure control versus tight glycaemic control. Data reproduced from UK Prospective Diabetes Study Group. Efficacy of atenolol and captopril in reducing risk of macrovascular and microvascular complications in type 2 diabetes: UKPDS 39. *BMJ* 1998;**317**:713–20. UK Prospective Diabetes Study Group. Tight blood pressure control and risk of macrovascular and microvascular complications in type 2 diabetes: UKPDS 38. *BMJ* 1998;**317**:703–13.

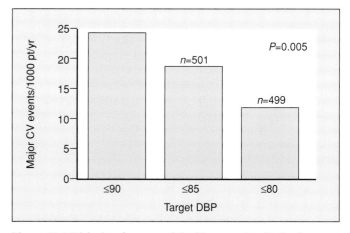

Figure 11.4 Diabetic sub-group of the Hypertension Optimal Treatment (HOT) Study. Reproduced with permission from Hansson L, Zanchetti A, Carruthers SG *et al*. Effects of intensive blood pressure lowering and low dose aspirin in patients with hypertension: principal results of the Hypertension Optimal Treatment randomised trial. *Lancet* 1998;**351**:1755–62.

Drugs in diabetic hypertensives	
ACE inhibitors	Protects kidney in IDDM
	Watch out for renal artery stenosis
Calcium channel blockers	Successful for NIDDM (HOT and SYST-Eur)
Thiazides	May worsen glucose tolerance and insulin resistance
Beta-blockers	Effective in NIDDM
Alpha-blockers	Metabolically neutral
	Lowers lipids
Angiotensin II receptor antagonists	Reduces proteinuria
	Trials underway

The recent MICRO-HOPE study (see box) confirms the beneficial effects of ACE inhibitors in diabetics, even beyond blood pressure lowering effects.

Despite several small surveillance studies suggesting that the calcium antagonists may be harmful, such a regimen was successful in reducing cardiovascular events in diabetics whose blood pressure was aggressively lowered in the HOT study. In the diabetic cohort of the HOT study, blood pressure lowering improved cardiovascular outcome and, importantly, there were 50% fewer cardiovascular endpoints when diastolic blood pressure was titrated beyond <90 mmHg to <80 mmHg. Dramatic survival benefits were also observed in the elderly diabetic cohort treated with calcium channel blockers in the SYST-Eur trial.

To summarise, the ACE inhibitors are probably the first choice for patients with both types of diabetes with proteinuria, with the calcium antagonists, beta-blockers and low dose diuretics also suitable in uncomplicated type 2 diabetes. ACE inhibitors have an antiproteinuric action and delay progression from microalbuminuria to overt nephropathy. They may possibly have a specific renoprotective action beyond blood pressure reduction in overt nephropathy, complicating type 2 diabetes. The threshold for intervention with antihypertensive therapy as >140/90 mmHg in type 2 diabetes. In addition, aspirin should possibly be offered to all patients with diabetes and hypertension once their blood pressure is controlled. Many type 2 diabetic people with hypertension will also require statin therapy to lower cholesterol for primary prevention because their estimated 10-year CHD risk is >30%.

MICRO-HOPE

Effects of ramipril on cardiovascular and microvascular outcomes in 3577 subjects with diabetes mellitus
Results of the HOPE study and MICRO-HOPE substudy. *Lancet* 2000; **355**: 253–9.

- In diabetics at risk for CVD, addition of ramipril to other effective therapies significantly reduces:
  CV death, strokes and MI
  total mortality
  revascularisation
  diabetic neuropathy
- The benefit is independent of the effect on BP

Ramipril was beneficial for cardiovascular events and overt nephropathy in people with diabetes.
The cardiovascular benefit was greater than that attributable to the decrease in blood pressure.

Further reading

- Mogensen CE. Combined high blood pressure and glucose in type 2 diabetes: double jeopardy. *BMJ* 1998;**317**:693–4.
- Orchard T. Diabetes: a time for excitement and concern. *BMJ* 1988;**317**:691–2.

12 Hypertension in pregnancy

In Western countries the hypertensive disorders of pregnancy are a major cause of maternal death with a risk of around 10 per million pregnancies. They are also the most common causes of fetal and neonatal death. Hypertension occurs at some stage in up to 10% of all pregnancies, and may be the first sign of impending pre-eclampsia, a potentially serious condition of the second half of pregnancy and the puerperium. Unfortunately, hypertension in pregnancy is still relatively poorly understood and there have been very few randomised controlled trials assessing its management. This chapter looks at different types of hypertension in pregnancy, the possible mechanisms, and the drug treatment of hypertension in pregnancy.

Classification of hypertension in pregnancy

There have been many attempts to classify the hypertensive disorders of pregnancy and none of them have been entirely satisfactory. This is partly because the diagnoses are often made in retrospect after the pregnancy is over. It is important to understand the different types of hypertension in pregnancy, not least because their prognosis differs widely.

Pre-existing hypertension

Probably the most benign category is pre-existing mild essential hypertension which, of course, becomes more common with advancing maternal age. Care must be taken to distinguish between chronic hypertension (defined as a blood pressure of >140/90 mmHg before 20 weeks' gestation) and very early pre-eclampsia. Elevated blood pressure before 20 weeks' gestation usually means that hypertension was pre-existing, before the pregnancy. This will commonly be "essential" but clinical evaluation is needed to exclude other causes such as renal disease, phaeochromocytoma, or aortic coarctation.

In these patients, blood pressure follows the normal pattern of pregnancy and may settle during the first trimester and then rise again later in the pregnancy. An apparent onset of hypertension after 20 weeks' gestation may reflect hypertension that was undetected prior to pregnancy, and disguised by the blood pressure fall that occurs in early to mid-pregnancy. All women with hypertension in pregnancy should have their blood pressure checked postnatally and if at six weeks postpartum it is greater than 140/90 mmHg, it is generally assumed the patient had chronic (but often undiagnosed) hypertension.

Secondary hypertension in pregnancy may be caused by renal diseases as well as the other conditions mentioned in previous chapters. It is important to exclude a diagnosis of phaeochromocytoma, which is associated with high maternal and fetal death rates.

Women with essential hypertension are at three-fold increased risk of developing pre-eclampsia or intrauterine growth restriction (IUGR). Management of pre-existing chronic hypertension should therefore include frequent blood

---

Problems with the classification of the hypertensive disorders of pregnancy

- Many women do not have their blood pressure measured before pregnancy and some may have had prior hypertension
- Blood pressure tends to settle in mid-pregnancy
- It is difficult to differentiate between mild pre-eclampsia and less ominous rises in blood pressure in late pregnancy
- It is impossible to predict whether rises in blood pressure in late pregnancy may proceed rapidly to severe pre-eclampsia
- Many women are opting for later pregnancies and may have mild essential hypertension

---

A simple classification of hypertensive disorders of pregnancy

1. Raised blood pressure (>140/90 mmHg) before 20 weeks' gestation
   a. Known chronic hypertension
      i. Essential
      ii. Renal (glomerulonephritis, pyelonephritis, polycystic kidney disease)
      iii. Renovascular (fibromuscular dysplasia)
      iv. Adrenal (phaeochromocytoma)
   b. Presumed chronic hypertension

2. Raised blood pressure (>140/90 mmHg) after 20 weeks' gestation
   a. Chronic hypertension
   b. Mild non-proteinuria pre-eclampsia
   c. Proteinuric pre-eclampsia
   d. Pre-eclampsia complicating chronic hypertension

In the above classification the term "pregnancy-induced hypertension" is abolished. Some of these would have chronic hypertension while others have mild early pre-eclampsia

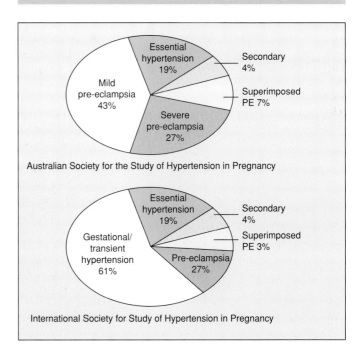

Figure 12.1 A comparison of two classifications of the hypertensive syndromes of pregnancy in 1183 consecutive pregnancies. PE = pre-eclampsia. Reproduced with permission from Brown MA, Biddle ML. *J Hypertens* 1997;**15**:1049–54.

pressure checks, preferably weekly at first, urinalysis, and an assessment of fetal growth. Early antenatal clinic referral should be made if the blood pressure exceeds 140/90 mmHg, there is new onset proteinuria, or if the mother is in a high risk category. Treatment may reduce the risk of progression to severe hypertension and hospital admissions. Firm evidence is not available on the optimal threshold for treatment, but treatment is essential at 160/100 mmHg, although many treat blood pressure at levels >140/90 mmHg.

Sadly there is no evidence that treating hypertension in early pregnancy can prevent the development of pre-eclampsia.

Pregnancy induced hypertension (PIH)

We prefer not to use this term as it implies that the mother was definitely normotensive prior to pregnancy but sustained a rise to 140/90 mmHg or more at some stage, but with no progression to florid pre-eclampsia. The current view is that PIH in the first half of pregnancy is probably really chronic, associated with obesity or a strong family history of hypertension. If the blood pressure rises de novo in the second half of pregnancy then PIH may really be very mild pre-eclampsia but it is impossible to be sure until after the pregnancy is over.

Pre-eclampsia

Pre-eclampsia occurrs in about 5% of first pregnancies and in about 15% of women with chronic hypertension. The criteria for the diagnosis of pre-eclampsia include: a rise in blood pressure of >15 mmHg diastolic or >30 mmHg systolic from early pregnancy, or diastolic blood pressure of >90 mmHg on two occasions four hours apart or >110 mmHg on one occasion and proteinuria (1+ is an indication for referral and >300 mg/24 hours is the criterion for diagnosis). Pre-eclampsia is seen in the early stages occasionally with normal blood pressures but proteinuria alone.

Women with pre-eclampsia generally have no symptoms and can only be detected by routine screening. When present, the most frequent symptoms are headache, visual disturbance (often "flashing lights"), vomiting, epigastric pain, and oedema (particularly facial oedema). These symptoms in conjunction with raised blood pressure and/or proteinuria require urgent referral and treatment. The prognosis of fully blown pre-eclampsia is much more sinister than the other hypertensive pregnancy syndromes.

Eclampsia

Full blown eclampsia is an obstetric emergency with a very high risk to the mother and fetus. Fortunately, this condition is rare in developed countries, occurring in about 1 in 500 pregnancies. In addition to hypertension and proteinuria, there is often gross oedema, and the more serious complications include cerebral oedema with hyperreflexia, convulsions, retinal haemorrhages and papilloedema, renal failure, pulmonary oedema, and disseminated intravascular coagulation. The clinical features of eclampsia may be of very rapid onset (that is, less than 24 hours in a previously fit mother). Women occasionally present with a convulsion with no hypertension or proteinuria. A first fit in the second half of pregnancy, with no other known cause, is highly suggestive of eclampsia.

High risk groups for pre-eclampsia

- Primigravidas
- Multigravida (>3 pregnancies) especially if new and recent sexual partner
- Teenage mothers
- Older mothers
- History of raised blood pressure
- Obesity—with problems of accurate blood pressure measurement
- Diabetic mothers
- Twin pregnancies
- Low social class/poor antenatal care
- Rhesus isoimmunisation
- Hydatiform mole
- Previous oral contraceptive hypertension (weak association)

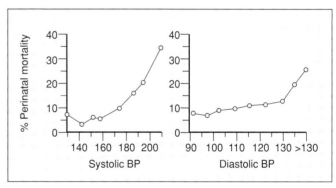

Figure 12.2 Perinatal mortality in pre-eclampsia (1960–69) in 4404 pregnancies. Reproduced with permission from Tervila L, Goecke C, Timonen S. Estimation of gestosis of pregnancy (EPH-Gestosis). *Acta Obstet Gynecol Scand* 1973;**52**:235–43.

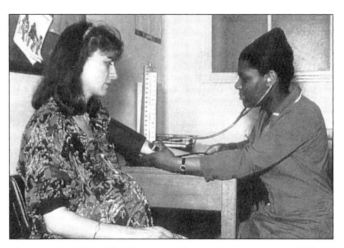

Figure 12.3 Taking blood pressure of a pregnant woman (published with permission from the patient)

Hypertension in pregnancy

Postpartum hypertension

In women with pre-eclampsia or even eclampsia, delivery of the baby and the placenta usually leads to a rapid fall in blood pressure. Occasionally the blood pressure may remain modestly raised for a few weeks postpartum. If this occurs, then it is most likely that the mother has pre-existing chronic hypertension.

Very rarely, in mothers with pre-eclampsia, blood pressure may rise sharply in the puerperium despite delivery of the placenta. The mechanism of this syndrome is uncertain but renal complications of pregnancy and of caesarean section should be excluded.

Women with pre-eclampsia have a higher risk of developing hypertension in later life and should therefore have annual blood pressure checks.

Aetiology of pre-eclampsia

Pre-eclampsia has several risk factors in common with hypertension in non-obstetric practice. It is now becoming clear that the origins of pre-eclampsia lie in abnormalities of implantation of the placenta in the first trimester where the damaged muscular coat and intima of the placental spiral arteries fail to demuscularise but instead undergo accelerated atherosclerosis ("acute atherosis") that further narrows and occludes the arterioles, resulting in a decrease in perfusion of the intervillous space. These lead to more acute ischaemia with vascular occlusions and placental infarctions, leading to fetal ischaemia and hypoxia, resulting in intrauterine growth retardation and, in severe cases, intrauterine death. It is unclear how this disease progresses to produce the syndrome of systemic hypertension and proteinuria.

The circulating renin-angiotensin system is certainly less activated than in normal pregnancies and, although there are disturbances of other vasoactive systems such as the kallikrein-kinin system and endothelin, the significance of these is not fully understood. It is probable that in pre-eclampsia there is increased pressure responsiveness to circulating angiotensin levels.

In severe pregnancy induced hypertension, platelets are both consumed and activated, leading to a coagulopathy, with activation of intravascular coagulation and fibrin deposition. The fibrinolytic system may also be involved, as increased maternal plasminogen activator inhibitor has been found. A few women develop a more serious complication, often referred to as the HELLP syndrome, which comprises haemolysis, elevated liver enzymes, and low platelets (H = haemolysis, EL = elevated liver enzymes. LP = low platelets). Maternal thrombocytopenia is significantly associated with maternal and perinatal mortality, with an increasing risk of eclampsia.

An immunological mechanism for eclampsia is supported by the reduced prevalence of pregnancy induced hypertension in women who have had prior full term pregnancy or blood transfusion. There is also an increased risk among users of contraceptives that prevent exposure to sperm, suggesting that pregnancy induced hypertension may be related to initial exposure of the patient to foreign antigen. The effects of pregnancy induced hypertension on organs other than the placenta are mediated by the hypertension or by the activation of components of the complement system, causing immune complex deposition on the renal basement membrane, thus allowing protein to leak into the urine.

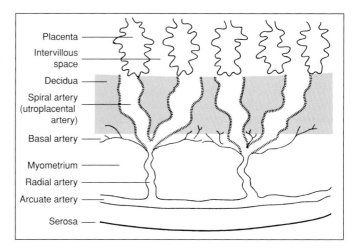

Figure 12.4 Diagram of the blood supply to the placenta in the third trimester. The spinal arteries (hatched) have been converted to utero-placental arteries from their origins from the radial arteries. (Reproduced with permission from Gerretsen G, Huisjes HJ, Elema JD. Morphological changes of the spiral arteries in the placental bed in relation to pre-eclampsia and fetal growth retardation. *Br J Obstet Gynaecol* 1981;**88**:876–81)

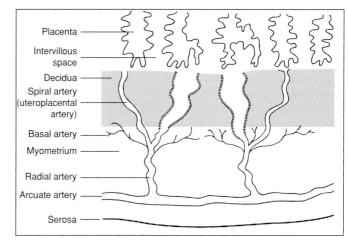

Figure 12.5 Diagram of the blood supply to the placenta in pre-eclampsia: the spiral arteries are either not converted to uteroplacental arteries (solid outlines) or, if they are, have been so converted only in their decidual segments (hatched outlines). (Reproduced with permission from Gerretson G, Huisjes HJ, Elema JD. Morphological changes of the spiral arteries in the placental bed in relation to pre-eclampsia and fetal growth retardation. *Br J Obstet Gynaecol* 1981;**88**:876–81)

Aetiology of pre-eclampsia—more common in:

- Advancing maternal age—paradoxically, there is also high incidence in young teenage mothers
- Those with a family history of pre-eclampsia
- Obese mothers
- Diabetics
- Low socioeconomic status
- First pregnancy
- Change of partner—the prevalence of pre-eclampsia falls in subsequent pregnancies by the same father, but pregnancies by different fathers are said to have the same rate as in primigravidas.
- Previous pre-eclampsia
- Idiopathic hypertension
- Chronic renal disease
- Systemic lupus erythematosus
- Multiple pregnancies or hydatiform mole
- Rhesus isoimmunisation

Management of hypertension in pregnancy

The hypertensive care of obstetric patients should probably start before they become pregnant. This entails monitoring the blood pressures of the young female population so that their baseline blood pressures are documented. Diastolic blood pressure should be measured at the disappearance of sounds (phase V) and not at muffling (phase IV), as recommended in the past.

Many women may be found to be mildly hypertensive, but treatment may not be required because these patients have a low absolute risk of developing cardiovascular complications. However, if treatment is instigated, ideally it should be with a drug that can be used safely in women who wish to become pregnant. The ACE inhibitors and the angiotensin receptor antagonists should be avoided if possible. If and when a woman becomes pregnant, these drugs, and also the beta-blockers (particularly atenolol) and thiazide diuretics, should be stopped, and if necessary, other agents substituted. However, evidence underpinning the choice of antihypertensive therapy in pregnancy is inadequate to make firm recommendations.

Mild hypertension in pregnancy with pressures below 150/100 mmHg, particularly if detected in the first 20 weeks of gestation, should usually not be treated with drugs. This is because the raised blood pressure is probably caused by mild essential hypertension, and there is evidence to suggest that these women have no increase in perinatal mortality, even though there is an increased risk of pre-eclampsia. These patients should, however, undergo basic investigation. If hypertension is more severe, then antihypertensive medication should be started, occasionally after admission to hospital for assessment. The development of proteinuria in association with hypertension in the second half of pregnancy implies a diagnosis of pre-eclampsia. These women should always be admitted to hospital for full assessment and control of their blood pressure. If pre-eclampsia develops near the end of the pregnancy, the optimum treatment is delivery of the baby while maintaining good blood pressure control.

There have only been a limited number of randomised controlled trials of the treatment of hypertensive disorders of pregnancy. A meta-analysis of those available was published in 1999, and this clarifies some points:

- The treatment of mild hypertension in early pregnancy does not prevent pre-eclampsia or IUGR.
- There is little information on the treatment of severe hypertension in early pregnancy, but this treatment is mainly to protect the mother from heart attack, angina, or stroke.
- Bed rest is of no value.
- The more aggressive treatment of hypertension in late pregnancy leads to a reduction of hospital admissions, preterm delivery, etc.
- There is no obvious optimum choice of drug(s) for severe hypertension in late pregnancy.

Hazards of hypertension in pregnancy

To the mother:
- Renal failure
- Stroke
- Eclamptic fits
- Hyperreflexia
- Hepatic failure
- Retinal detachment
- Papilloedema, retinal haemorrhage
- Irritability
- HELLP syndrome

To the baby:
- Placental insufficiency
- Placental infarctions
- Intrauterine growth retardation
- Intrauterine death
- Necessity of early delivery

Blood pressure measurement in pregnancy

- Most automatic and semiautomatic blood pressure monitoring systems have not been validated in pregnancy. BP checks using conventional mercury manometers should be carried out at least once in all mothers
- Diastolic blood pressures should be taken at phase five (disappearance of sounds)
- The measurement of blood pressure with mothers lying on their side is not known to be useful
- Where possible blood pressure should be measured with the patient seated
- A minimum of two BP readings should be taken at each antenatal clinic visit
- A conventional "adult" and a larger "alternative adult" should be available in all clinics

---

Table 12.1 Laboratory tests in hypertension in pregnancy

Test	Rationale
Full blood count	• Haemoconcentration is found in pre-eclampsia and is an indicator of severity • Decreased platelet count suggests severe pre-eclampsia
Blood film	• Microangiopathic haemolytic anaemia may occur in severe pre-eclampsia/eclampsia
Urinalysis	• If dipstick proteinuria of 1+ or more, a quantitative measurement of 24-hour protein excretion is required • Hypertensive pregnant women with proteinuria should be considered to have pre-eclampsia until proven otherwise
Serum uric acid	• Raised in pre-eclampsia/elampsia
Serum albumin	• Levels may be decreased even with mild proteinuria, perhaps due to capillary leak or hepatic involvement in pre-eclampsia
Serum urea and creatinine	• Usually low in pregnancy. "Normal" non-pregnancy levels may indicate renal impairment
Liver function tests	• Aspartate and alanine transaminase levels rise in the HELLP syndrome

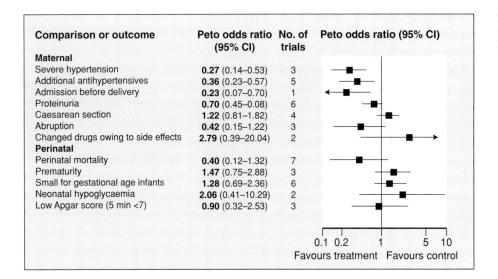

Comparison or outcome	Peto odds ratio (95% CI)	No. of trials	Peto odds ratio (95% CI)
Maternal			
Severe hypertension	**0.27** (0.14–0.53)	3	
Additional antihypertensives	**0.36** (0.23–0.57)	5	
Admission before delivery	**0.23** (0.07–0.70)	1	
Proteinuria	**0.70** (0.45–0.08)	6	
Caesarean section	**1.22** (0.81–1.82)	4	
Abruption	**0.42** (0.15–1.22)	3	
Changed drugs owing to side effects	**2.79** (0.39–20.04)	2	
Perinatal			
Perinatal mortality	**0.40** (0.12–1.32)	7	
Prematurity	**1.47** (0.75–2.88)	3	
Small for gestational age infants	**1.28** (0.69–2.36)	6	
Neonatal hypoglycaemia	**2.06** (0.41–10.29)	2	
Low Apgar score (5 min <7)	**0.90** (0.32–2.53)	3	

0.1 0.2 1 5 10
Favours treatment   Favours control

Figure 12.6 Antihypertensive treatment in pregnancy for mild chronic hypertension.

Comparison or outcome	Peto odds ratio (95% CI)	No. of trials	Peto odds ratio (95% CI)
Maternal			
Severe hypertension	**0.36** (0.26–0.49)	13	
Additional antihypertensives	**0.39** (0.26–0.59)	6	
Admission before delivery	**0.45** (0.30–0.67)	4	
Proteinuria at delivery	**0.67** (0.51–0.89)	12	
Caesarean section	**0.95** (0.76–1.20)	4	
Abruption	**2.50** (0.76–8.21)	7	
Changed drugs owing to side effects	**2.59** (0.93–7.20)	8	
Maternal mortality	**7.20** (0.14–363.10)	3	
Perinatal			
Perinatal mortality	**0.68** (0.36–1.25)	15	
Prematurity	**0.97** (0.72–1.31)	7	
Small for gestational age infants	**1.35** (0.96–1.88)	9	
Admission to special care baby unit	**1.04** (0.77–1.40)	7	
Neonatal jaundice	**0.53** (0.22–1.28)	2	
Neonatal hypoglycaemia	**0.76** (0.37–1.57)	3	
Neonatal bradycardia	**2.14** (1.09–4.20)	3	
Low Apgar score (5 min <7)	**0.56** (0.17–1.87)	3	
Respiratory distress syndrome	**0.27** (0.13–0.54)	5	

0.1 0.2 1 5 10
Favours treatment   Favours control

Figure 12.7 Antihypertensive treatment in late pregnancy. Figures 12.4 and 12.5 reproduced with permission from Magee LA, Ornstein MP, von Dadelszen P. Management of hypertension in pregnancy. *BMJ* 1999;**318**:1332–6.

Blood pressure reduction in pregnancy

Non-pharmacological manoeuvres to reduce blood pressure in pregnancy have not been extensively addressed. Strict bed rest is not indicated and may be harmful, but reduced physical activity may be appropriate. Salt restriction is of no value and may even be harmful.

Drug treatment when indicated must take into consideration any potential effects of antihypertensive drugs on the fetus. For example, angiotensin converting enzyme (ACE) inhibitors are absolutely contraindicated in pregnancy because they have been associated with congenital abnormalities, growth retardation, oligohydramnios, renal failure, hypotension and intrauterine death in the fetus. There is no information on the angiotensin receptor antagonists, so these drugs must not be used. Women who conceive while taking these agents should stop them as soon as pregnancy is diagnosed. They can however be reassured that with early discontinuation, there appears to be no excess risk to the fetus.

Methyldopa remains the antihypertensive drug of choice for idiopathic hypertension or pre-eclampsia because of its long and extensive use without reports of serious adverse

Average BP recordings when treatment initiated in the antenatal hypertension clinic at the City Hospital, Birmingham 1980–1999 (unpublished observations)

- 1980–1985
  av SBP 153 (SD 15.7)
  av DBP 98 (SD 8.7)
- 1985–1989
  av SBP 151 (SD 16)
  av DBP 101 (SD 8.7)
- 1990–1995
  av SBP 155 (SD 18.2)
  av DBP 101 (SD 8.4)
- 1995–1999
  av SBP 161 (SD 15.3)
  av DBP 104 (SD 9.4)

effects on the fetus. However methyldopa can cause sedation and lethargy and possibly postnatal depression. Calcium antagonists (especially nifedipine) and the vasodilator hydralazine are commonly used as second line drugs. The calcium channel blocker, nifedipine, has been used safely, but only in severe resistant hypertension in pregnancy. The alpha-blockers are probably safe but the newer ones, such as doxazosin, have yet to undergo formal testing.

Labetalol (combined alpha- and beta-blocker) is also widely used in pregnancy, either as an adjunct to or as an alternative to methyldopa. Information is now available to suggest that atenolol and propranolol, particularly before 28 weeks' gestation, may be associated with reduced fetal blood flow and smaller babies. The other beta-blockers, such as oxprenolol and pindolol, may be safer but only limited data are available.

Diuretics are not generally used to treat hypertension in pregnancy. They slightly reduce intravascular volume which in pre-eclampsia is already reduced. This may cause a fall in utero-placental blood flow. Nevertheless, meta-analysis of controlled trials of diuretics has shown a reduced incidence of pre-eclampsia, although no benefit was shown on fetal outcome.

In the emergency management of hypertension in mothers with severe pre-eclampsia or eclampsia, intravenous and intramuscular drugs may be required such as hydralazine or labetalol, together with anticonvulsants and magnesium sulphate. These patients should be admitted to well equipped and staffed obstetric units with adequate facilities for intensive neonatal care.

Aspirin

The value of low dose aspirin in high risk pregnancies was tested in the CLASP trial. The latter was largely negative but there was some evidence that aspirin was beneficial in some very high risk pregnancies, up until about three weeks before a planned delivery. There is as yet no information on its use in mothers with hypertension alone. It is probably best to reserve it for use in those cases where there has been a previous history of intrauterine death, stillbirth, or intrauterine growth retardation.

Conclusion

Hypertensive women who plan pregnancy, or who become pregnant while on antihypertensive treatment, should be advised to change their therapy to one of the drugs recommended for the treatment of hypertension in pregnancy. It is usual to switch from such agents back to the previous antihypertensive regimen after delivery. There has, over the past 10 years, been a tendency increasingly to withhold drug therapy in mothers with blood pressures below 150/100 mmHg. The decision to give drugs to pregnant women should probably only be made by highly qualified obstetricians or physicians with special experience of managing hypertension in pregnancy.

	n	Birth Weight	Ponderal index Wt (kg)/length (m)^3 $\times 10^4$
Untreated	91	3.07	23.7
Atenolol	78	2.37	22.2
Other monotherapies	53	2.76	23.5
Multiple drugs	90	2.22	22.6

Figure 12.8 The effects of atenolol on birth weight in the City Hospital Birmingham Antenatal Hypertension Clinic. Lydakis C, Lip GYH, Beevers M, Beevers DG. Atenolol and fetal growth in pregnancies complicated by hypertension. *Am J Hypertens* 1999;**12**:541–7.

Drug treatments for hypertension in pregnancy

Contraindicated:
- ACE inhibitors
- Calcium channel blockers in mild hypertension
- Thiazides
- Atenolol, propranolol

Probably safe:
- Methyldopa, particularly in asthmatic mothers
- Alpha-blockers
- Some beta-blockers, e.g., labetalol, oxprenolol, pindolol
- Nifedipine in severe cases

Emergency:
- Intravenous and intramuscular drugs, e.g., hydralazine, labetalol
- Anticonvulsants
- Magnesium sulfate

Further reading

- Broughton Pipkin F. The hypertensive disorders of pregnancy. *BMJ* 1995;**311**:609–13.
- Churchill DC, Beevers DG. *Hypertension in pregnancy*. London. BMJ Books, 1999.
- National High Blood Pressure Education Program Working Group Report on High Blood Pressure in Pregnancy. *Am J Obstet Gynecol* 1990;**163**:1689–1712.
- Sibai BM. Treatment of hypertension in pregnant women. *New Engl J Med* 1996;**335**:257–65.

13   Hypertension in primary care

There is firm evidence that the accurate detection, assessment, and treatment of hypertensive patients is a well validated medical intervention that leads to a significant reduction in the number of strokes and heart attacks. Sadly, however, there is also evidence that a very large number of hypertensive patients are not receiving the treatment they need as a result of deficiencies in the methods of delivery of health care. The "rule of halves" (an expression first coined in the 1960s) still prevails unless special efforts are made. Surveys revealing incomplete detection, treatment and control of hypertension indicate a serious failure to implement the knowledge we have, although there has been some improvement in recent years. A WHO-WHL (World Health Organisation—World Hypertension) audit project in several European countries showed that no more than 29% of all treated hypertensive patients had attained adequate blood pressure control, and there was a failure to implement non-pharmacological measures to reduce blood pressure and cardiovascular risk. A study from Australia showed that hypertensive patients were no more knowledgeable than normotensive controls about hypertension, and 70% of patients expressed a desire for more information about their condition.

As a result of the Hypertension Optimal Treatment (HOT) trial, we now know that the target in treated hypertensives is to reduce the blood pressure to below 140/85 mmHg. With this new target, the Health Survey for England has revealed that less than 10% of hypertensive patients are receiving optimal treatment and blood pressure control.

As the vast majority of hypertensive patients do not (and should not) attend hospital, it is clear that the management of millions of mildly hypertensive patients can only be achieved within the context of the primary health care team. The systems for delivery of primary health care differ among nations, but the principles remain the same everywhere.

In the United Kingdom the routine measurement of blood pressure in all adults is now considered to be an integral part of good medical care. All British citizens have a named general practitioner or family doctor. Evidence that blood pressures are being measured routinely is now being demanded by health care administrators and suitable clinical audit programmes are being devised.

In addition, there has been an expansion in the number of nurse practitioners working in close collaboration with general practitioners. These nurses can, with adequate training, organise the detection, management, and follow up of most hypertensive patients.

Screening

As hypertension is usually an asymptomatic condition, clearly some form of screening is necessary to detect cases. Although dedicated screening units can help, these are not, in general, to be encouraged because they do not have the appropriate methods of follow up and are often organised on a "one-off" basis. The ongoing screening of asymptomatic patients for high blood pressure should, therefore, take place within the context of primary health care.

As between 70% and 80% of the population are likely to visit a doctor for some reason at least once in three years, it is

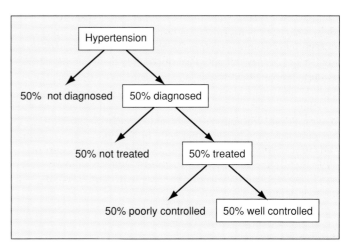

Figure 13.1 The "rule of halves" – what happens to hypertensive patients if special efforts are not made to improve screening, prescribing, and blood pressure control

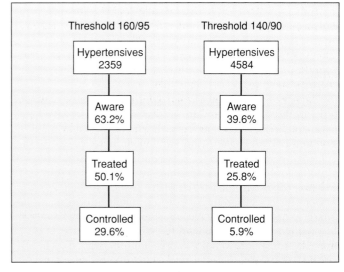

Figure 13.2 Health Survey for England 1994 – Proportions aware, treated, and controlled if blood pressure thresholds were 160/95 and 140/90 mmHg. Reproduced with permission from Colhoun HM, Dong W, Paulter NR. Blood pressure screening, management and control in England: results from the health survey for England 1994. *J Hypertens* 1998;**16**:747–52.

It does not matter how severe the hypertension was at first presentation. What does matter is the quality of control of the blood pressure at follow up preferable that screening should take place at this time. This system, referred to as "opportunist screening", has been demonstrated to be effective in general practice in both a city centre and rural environment. All patients who visit their general practitioners should have their blood pressure checked if they have not attended for more than 12 months. All those whose blood pressures exceed 140/90 mmHg should be advised that their blood pressures are not quite normal and recalled for re-examination a few weeks later. The nurse practitioner is the best member of the health care team to arrange this procedure.

Rescreening

The BHS recommends rescreening previously normotensive adults at all ages every five years but annual rescreening for people with previously raised readings that have settled as well as those who are "high normal".

Assessment

If, after four consultations, with two readings on each occasion, the systolic blood pressure still exceeds 160 mmHg and the diastolic blood pressure 90 mmHg, then more detailed assessment is necessary. In patients with evidence of target organ damage (transient ischaemic attack (TIA), stroke, angina, previous myocardial infarction) or concurrent diabetes mellitus, the threshold should be 140/90 mmHg. All such patients should undergo a routine Dipstix urine test, a single blood test to measure renal function and serum lipid levels, and an ECG to assess left ventricular size.

The optimum method of managing these patients is set out in the guidelines suggested by the British Hypertension Society in 1999. Similar useful guidelines have also been produced in New Zealand and the United States.

High risk groups

Certain patient groups should be sought out specifically rather than waiting for them to attend for some other reason. It is probable that special appointments should be sent to such patients. This "selective screening" should be conducted in patients who are at particular risk of developing hypertension or its vascular complications, including those shown in the box.

Medical records

If chronic diseases such as hypertension are to be managed efficiently, then it is necessary to have good medical records. The increasing sophistication of computer software means that this can be achieved without difficulty. However, even the old fashioned records system still used in some health centres in the UK (the Lloyd George envelope) can be adapted for the management of hypertension.

Computerised systems can render clinical audit very feasible so that clinicians can investigate how frequently they reach the target for the detection of hypertension, the use of non-pharmacological treatments, and the introduction of blood pressure lowering drugs and the achievement of blood pressure targets.

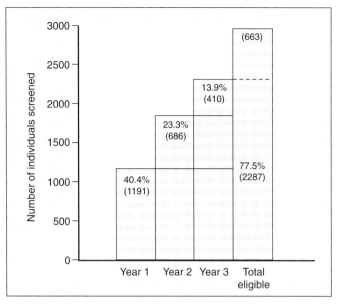

Figure 13.3 "Opportunistic screening". General practice case detection of hypertension in men aged 35–69 years: taken from records of six general practitioners. Reproduced from Barber JH, Beevers DG, Fife R *et al*. Blood pressure screening and supervision in general practice. *BMJ* 1979;**i**:843–6.

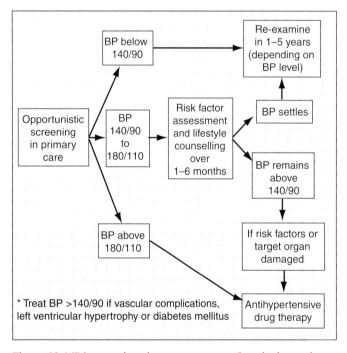

Figure 13.4 Triage or three-box management of newly detected hypertension in primary care

High risk groups

- Patients with a previous vascular complication of hypertension
- Patients with diabetes mellitus or hyperlipidaemia or smokers
- Patients with other systemic diseases including renal disease, polyarteritis, systemic lupus erythematosus, and peripheral vascular disease
- Pregnant women
- Patients with renal impairment
- People with a family history of hypertension, heart attack, or stroke

HYPERTENSION COOPERATION CARD

Name: *Thomas Smith* DOB 16 / 02 / 38

Address: *47 Anstrother Street*

Post Code *W27 9BU*

General Practitioner: *Dr Antrobus*

Date diagnosed hypertensive 16 / 2 / 94

Cigarette smoker No / (Yes) Quantity *20/d*

Advice:
(1) avoid being overweight
(2) moderate alcohol consumption
(3) restrict salt intake
(4) show this card to all doctors and nurses who look after you
(5) always bring your tablets when consulting your doctor or nurse
(6) don't stop taking tablets unless advised to by your doctor or nurse
(7) your target blood pressure is below 140/80 mmHg

Date	16/2/94	19/3/94	17/5/94	21/7/94	19/10/94	17/11/94	12/1/95	6/5/95	19/8/95	27/11/95
B.P.1	172/106	170/100	168/100	152/92	156/94	154/90	138/84	136/82	132/84	134/82
PULSE	98	52								
B.P.2	168/98	168/98	172/98	148/90	152/92	152/94	134/80	132/78	135/85	128/80
URINE	NAD									
WEIGHT kg st lb	84.2	84.0	82.1	81.6	82.0	82.2	84.0	82.4	81.0	80.2
DRUG 1 *Bendrofluazide*			Start 2.5mg	2.5mg	Stop					
DRUG 2 *Lisinopril*					Start 10mg	Increase 20mg	20mg	20mg	20mg	20mg
DRUG 3										
DRUG 4										
DRUG 5										
DRUG 6 *Simvastatin*							Start 10mg	10mg	Increase 20mg	20mg
SERUM UREA	6.2					6.0				
SERUM POTASSIUM	4.2									
SERUM CHOLESTEROL	7.1									
NEXT VISIT	1/12	2/12	2/12	3/12	1/12	2/12	3/12	3/12	3/12	3/12
DOCTOR'S SIGNATURE	RA	AO	RA	RA	RA	RA	RA	RA	RA	AO

Figure 13.5 An example of a patient held hypertension cooperation card

Quality of care and audit

The quality of care of hypertensive patients might be enhanced by improved screening or case-finding; the use of computer based systems and protocols to support clinical decision making; workshops on hypertension for general practitioners and practice nurses; clinical audit; improved doctor-patient or nurse-patient communication; and increased patient education.

General practices or primary care groups should develop protocols for hypertension management that cover: the screening policy; initial evaluation and investigation; implementation of non-pharmacological measures; formal estimation of cardiovascular risk; treatment policy for antihypertensive drugs, aspirin and statins; treatment targets; policy for follow up; and methods for identifying and recalling patients who drop out of follow up. Written information should be available for patients about hypertension and its treatment, and on non-pharmacological measures to reduce blood pressure and cardiovascular risk. The practice policy should detail those aspects of management that are in the province of the practice nurse and of the doctor, and the indications and procedure for passing management from nurse to doctor or vice versa.

The 1999 British Hypertension Society Guidelines recommended that implementation of the practice policy should be audited periodically, especially because several aspects of hypertension management lend themselves readily to audit procedures that are objective and reasonably simple.

Specialist referral

About 10% of hypertensive patients in primary health care have underlying causes for their high blood pressure or have very severe or resistant hypertension. Most of these patients need referral to a specialist centre for detailed investigation and management.

Examples of audit recommended by the British Hypertension Society

- The proportion of all adults in the practice who have had a blood pressure measurement in the last five years
- The proportion of all hypertensives given non-pharmacological advice
- The proportion of all hypertensives given antihypertensive therapy
- The proportion of hypertensives receiving antihypertensive therapy who have suboptimal control; i.e., BP levels >150 mmHg systolic and >90 mmHg diastolic
- The proportion of patients lost from follow up; or of treated patients who have not been reviewed within the last six months
- The use of aspirin and statins by those who require secondary prevention; or their use when indicated for primary prevention; i.e., when the estimated 10-year CHD risk is >5% (aspirin) or >30% per year (statins)

90% of hypertensive patients can be managed by the primary health care team without hospital referral

Keeping up to date

The vast majority of hypertensive patients can be managed exclusively in the primary care context. It is important, however, that primary care nurses and clinicians are kept in touch with the new information that is continually becoming available (several important papers on the treatment of hypertension have been published since 1991). It is important that public health physicians and administrators make special efforts to ensure that the health care providers are up to date and are achieving the appropriate targets.

It was commented some years ago by the distinguished general practitioner Julian Tudor-Hart that when a premature stroke occurs in a hypertensive patient, then the possibility that there has been clinical neglect should be considered. We now have reliable evidence that almost all strokes, which are caused by hypertension, can be prevented with accurate antihypertensive treatment. There is also evidence that a substantial impact can be made on the incidence of coronary heart disease. The prime responsibility for the administration of this validated health care rests in general practice, but considerable changes are necessary in the way that clinicians practice medicine (particularly for chronic diseases). It is the responsibility of general practitioners to seek out people who might have hypertension rather than waiting for them to present at a late stage of their disease, when they become clinically unwell with cardiovascular complications. General practitioners are thus responsible for the health of all the patients allocated to them and not just to those presenting with clinical illness.

Hypertension clinics

- Many general practitioners have established dedicated hypertension clinics to achieve efficient ongoing of their patients
- These clinics can best be run by appropriately trained and supervised nurse practitioners with well devised computerised protocols and medical records
- There is evidence that nurses can obtain better results than doctors in reducing blood pressure

Further reading

- British Cardiac Society, British Hyperlipidaemia Association, British Hypertension Society, British Diabetic Association. Joint British Recommendations on prevention of coronary heart disease in clinical practice: summary. *BMJ* 2000;**320**:705–8.
- Ramsay LE, Williams B, Johnston GD *et al*. British Hypertension Society guidelines for hypertension management 1999: summary. *BMJ* 1999;**319**:630–5.
- Ramsay LE, Williams B, Johnston GD *et al*. Guidelines for the management of hypertension: report of the third working party of the British Hypertension Society. *J Hum Hypertens* 1999;**13**:569–92.
- Taylor FC, Ebrahim S. Prevention of cardiovascular disease in hypertensive patients in general practice: improving the quality of care. *Br J Cardiol* 1997;**4**:331–5.
- Whitfield M, Hughes A. Hypertension management in general practice. *J Roy Soc Med* 1997;**90**:12–15.

Appendix A: Coronary risk prediction chart

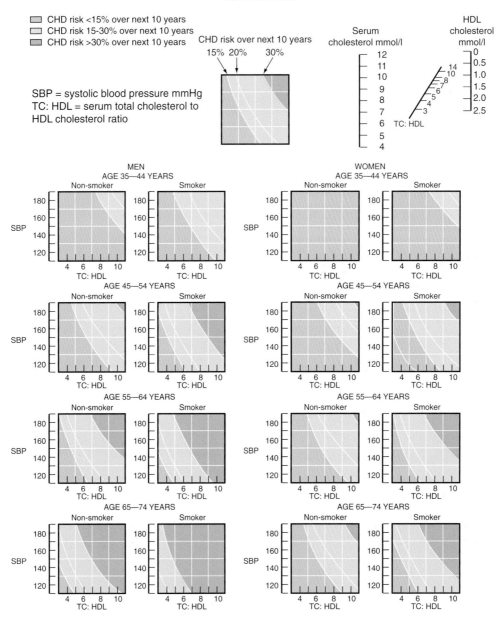

NO DIABETES

CHD risk <15% over next 10 years
CHD risk 15-30% over next 10 years
CHD risk >30% over next 10 years

CHD risk over next 10 years
15% 20% 30%

SBP = systolic blood pressure mmHg
TC: HDL = serum total cholesterol to HDL cholesterol ratio

Serum cholesterol mmol/l

HDL cholesterol mmol/l

How to use the Coronary Risk Prediction Chart for Primary Prevention

These charts are for estimating coronary heart disease (CHD) risk (non fatal MI and coronary death) for individuals who have not developed symptomatic CHD or other major atherosclerotic disease.

The use of these charts is not appropriate for patients who have existing disease which already puts them at high risk. Such diseases are:

- CHD or other major atherosclerotic disease
- Familial hypercholesterolaemia or other inherited dyslipidaemia
- Established hypertension (systolic BP > 160 mmHg and/or diastolic BP > 100 mmHg) or associated target organ damage
- Diabetes mellitus with associated target organ damage
- Renal dysfunction

- To estimate an individuals absolute 10 year risk of developing CHD find the table for their gender, diabetes (yes/no), smoking status (smoker/non-smoker) and age. Within this square define the level of risk according to systolic blood pressure and the ratio of total cholesterol to HDL cholesterol. If there is no HDL cholesterol then assume this is 1.0 mmol/l and then the lipid scale can be used for total cholesterol alone.
- High risk individuals are defined as those whose 10 year CHD risk exceeds 15% (equivalent to a *cardiovascular* risk of 20% over the same period). As a minimum those at highest risk (≥ 30% red) should be targeted and treated now, and as resources allow others with a risk of > 15% (orange) should be progressively targeted.

DIABETES

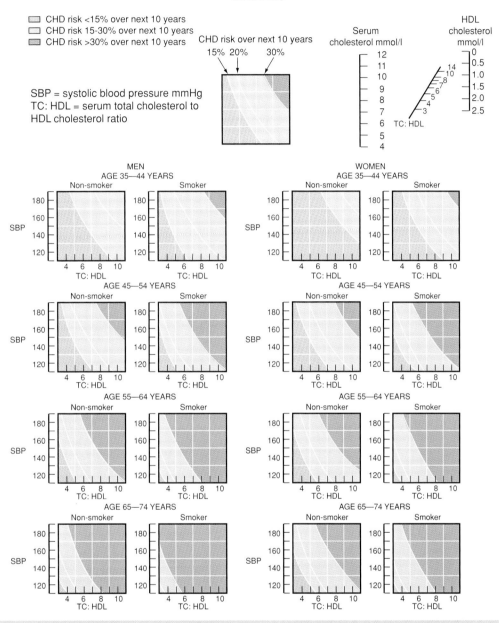

☐ CHD risk <15% over next 10 years
☐ CHD risk 15-30% over next 10 years
▨ CHD risk >30% over next 10 years

SBP = systolic blood pressure mmHg
TC: HDL = serum total cholesterol to
HDL cholesterol ratio

CHD risk over next 10 years
15% 20% 30%

Serum cholesterol mmol/l

HDL cholesterol mmol/l

MEN

AGE 35—44 YEARS

AGE 45—54 YEARS

AGE 55—64 YEARS

AGE 65—74 YEARS

WOMEN

AGE 35—44 YEARS

AGE 45—54 YEARS

AGE 55—64 YEARS

AGE 65—74 YEARS

- Smoking status should reflect lifetime exposure to tobacco and not simply tobacco use at the time of risk assessment.

- The initial blood pressure and the first random (non fasting) total cholesterol and HDL cholesterol can be used to estimate an individuals risk. However, the decision on using drug therapy should be based on repeat risk factor measurements over a period of time. The chart should not be used to estimate the risk after treatment of hyperlipidaemia or blood pressure has been initiated.

- CHD risk is higher than indicated in the charts for
  - Those with a family history of premature CHD (men <55 years and women <65 years) which increases the risk by a factor of approximately 1.5.
  - Those with raised triglyceride levels
  - Those who are not diabetic but have impaired glucose tolerance.
  - Women with premature menopause.

  - As the person approaches the next age category. As risk increases exponentially with age the risk will be closer to the higher decennium for the last four years of each decade.

- In ethnic minorities the risk chart should be used with caution as it has not been validated in these populations.

- The estimates of CHD risk from the chart are based on groups of people and in managing an *individual* the physician also has to use clinical judgement in deciding how intensively to intervene on lifestyle and whether or not to use drug therapies.

- An individual can be shown on the chart the direction in which the risk of CHD can be reduced by changing smoking status, blood pressure or cholesterol.

Index

Page numbers in **bold** type refer to figures and those in *italic* refer to tables or boxed material.

Index

Index

Index

Titles in the ABC series from BMJ Books

ABC of AIDS (4th edition)
Edited by Michael W Adler

ABC of Alcohol (3rd edition)
Alex Paton

ABC of Allergies
Edited by Stephen R Durham

ABC of Antenatal Care (3rd edition)
Geoffrey Chamberlain

ABC of Arterial and Venous Disease
Richard Donnelly and Nick JM London

ABC of Asthma (4th edition)
John Rees and Dipak Kanabar

ABC of Atrial Fibrillation
Edited by Gregory Y H Lip

ABC of Brain Stem Death (2nd edition)
C Pallis and D H Harley

ABC of Breast Diseases (2nd edition)
Edited by Michael Dixon

ABC of Child Abuse (3rd edition)
Edited by Roy Meadow

ABC of Clinical Genetics (revised 2nd edition)
Helen Kingston

ABC of Clinical Haematology
Drew Provan and Andrew Henson

ABC of Colorectal Diseases (2nd edition)
Edited by D J Jones

ABC of Dermatology (3rd edition)
Paul K Buxton

ABC of Dermatology (Hot Climates edition)
Paul K Buxton

ABC of Diabetes (4th edition)
Peter Watkins

ABC of Emergency Radiology
Edited by D Nicholson and P Driscoll

ABC of Eyes (3rd edition)
P T Khaw and A R Elkington

ABC of Healthy Travel (5th edition)
Eric Walker, Glyn Williams, Fiona Raeside and Lorna Calvert

ABC of Heart Failure
Christopher R Gibbs, Michael K Davies and Gregory YH Lip

ABC of Hypertension (4th edition)
Gareth Beevers, Gregory YH Lip and Eoin O'Brien

ABC of Intensive Care
Edited by Mervyn Singer and Ian Grant

ABC of Labour Care
G Chamberlain, P Steer and L Zander

ABC of Major Trauma (3rd edition)
Edited by David Skinner and Peter Driscoll

ABC of Medical Computing
Nicholas Lee and Andrew Millman

ABC of Mental Health
Edited by Teifion Davies and T K J Craig

ABC of Monitoring Drug Therapy
J K Aronson, M Hardman and D J M Reynolds

ABC of Nutrition (3rd edition)
A Stewart Truswell

ABC of One to Seven (4th edition)
H B Valman

ABC of Oral Health
Crispian Scully

ABC of Otolaryngology (4th edition)
Harold Ludman

ABC of Palliative Care
Edited by Marie Fallon and Bill O'Neill

ABC of Resuscitation (4th edition)
Edited by M C Colquhoun, A J Handley and T R Evans

ABC of Rheumatology (2nd edition)
Edited by Michael L Snaith

ABC of Sexual Health
Edited by John Tomlinson

ABC of Sexually Transmitted Diseases (4th edition)
Michael W Adler

ABC of Spinal Cord Injury (3rd edition)
David Grundy and Andrew Swain

ABC of Sports Medicine (2nd edition)
Edited by G McLatchie, M Harries, C Williams and J King

ABC of Transfusion (3rd edition)
Edited by Marcela A Contreras

ABC of Urology
Chris Dawson and Hugh Whitfield

ABC of Vascular Diseases
Edited by John Wolfe

ABC of Work Related Disorders
Edited by David Snashall

The First Year of Life (4th edition)
H B Valman

To order, please contact BMJ Bookshop, PO Box 295, London WC1H 9TE, UK
Tel: +44 (0)20 7383 6244   **Fax**: +44 (0)20 7383 6455   **Email**: orders@bmjbookshop.com

U.W.E.L. LEARNING RESOURCES